Diabetes Care
at a Glance

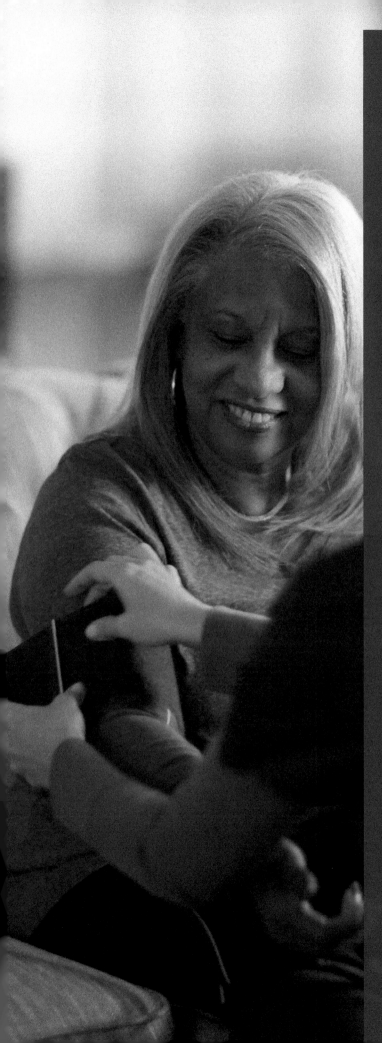

Diabetes Care
at a Glance

Edited by

Anne Phillips
PhD, MSc, NTF, RNT, QN, BSc Hons,
NDN, RGN
Professor in Diabetes Care
Programme Lead for Advancing Diabetes Care
Birmingham City University, Edgbaston
Birmingham, UK

Series Editor: Ian Peate

WILEY Blackwell

This first edition first published 2023
© 2023 by John Wiley & Sons Ltd

The right of Anne Phillips to be identified as the author of the editorial material in this work has been asserted in accordance with law.

Registered Offices
John Wiley & Sons, Inc., 111 River Street, Hoboken, NJ 07030, USA
John Wiley & Sons Ltd, The Atrium, Southern Gate, Chichester, West Sussex, PO19 8SQ, UK

For details of our global editorial offices, customer services, and more information about Wiley products visit us at www.wiley.com.

Wiley also publishes its books in a variety of electronic formats and by print-on-demand. Some content that appears in standard print versions of this book may not be available in other formats.

Library of Congress Cataloging-in-Publication Data applied for
Paperback ISBN: 9781119841265

Cover Image: © John Fedele/Getty Images
Cover design by Wiley

Set in 9.5/11.5 pt MinionPro by Straive, Pondicherry, India
Printed and bound by CPI Group (UK) Ltd, Croydon, CR0 4YY

C9781119841265_040123

This textbook is for every practitioner who would like to learn more about caring for people with diabetes and may see this specialism as an exciting career prospect to follow – we encourage you and thank you.

This textbook is also dedicated to Sandra Dudley, a dedicated Diabetes Specialist Nurse who spent her career working with people with diabetes and latterly introducing insulin pump therapy back into the UK. Sandra made a substantial difference to every person with type 1 diabetes she met and cared for – thank you Sandra.

Contents

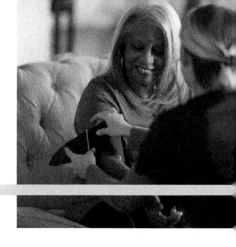

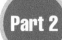

Contributors

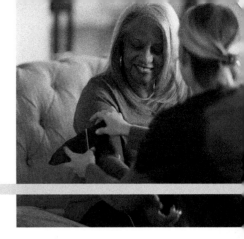

Julie Cropper [Chapter 43]
Genetic Diabetes Nurse/North East and Yorkshire GMSA Nurse Lead, St James's University Hospital, Leeds Teaching Hospitals NHS Trust, Leeds, UK

Adele Farnsworth [Chapters 37, 38]
Senior Diabetic Retinal Screener and Grader, University Hospitals Birmingham NHS Foundation Trust, Birmingham, UK

Carole Gelder [Chapter 26]
Children's Diabetes Specialist Nurse and Clinical Educator, Leeds Children's Hospital, Leeds and Senior Lecturer, Birmingham City University, Birmingham, UK

Peter Jennings [Chapters 2, 13, 17, 19, 20]
Senior Lecturer for Advancing Diabetes Care, Birmingham City University, Birmingham, UK

Aoife Kelleher [Chapter 43]
Consultant in Paediatric Diabetes, Leeds Children's Hospital, Leeds, UK

Angela Phillips [Chapter 39]
Diabetes Specialist Nurse, University Hospitals Birmingham NHS Foundation Trust, Birmingham, UK

Anne Phillips [Chapters 1, 3, 4, 6, 10–13, 21, 22, 29, 34, 35, 41, 42, 44, 45]
Professor in Diabetes Care, Programme Lead for Advancing Diabetes Care, Birmingham City University, Edgbaston, Birmingham, UK

Paul Pipe-Thomas [Chapters 5, 7, 9]
Clinical Specialist Dietitian for Diabetes, Rotherham NHS Foundation Trust, Rotherham, UK

Jayne Robbie [Chapters 30–33, 40]
Senior Lecturer in Advancing Diabetes Care, Birmingham City University and Specialist Podiatrist, University Hospitals Birmingham NHS Trust, Birmingham, UK

Susan Sayapi [Chapter 36]
Diabetes and Renal Specialist Nurse, University Hospitals Birmingham NHS Foundation Trust, Birmingham, UK

Theresa Smyth [Chapters 27, 28, 46]
Nurse Consultant in Diabetes, University Hospitals Birmingham NHS Foundation Trust and Honorary Visiting Professor, Birmingham City University, Birmingham, UK

Martha Stewart [Chapters 8, 14–16, 18, 23–25]
Senior Lecturer in Advancing Diabetes Care, Birmingham City University, and Diabetes Clinical Nurse Specialist, University Hospitals Birmingham NHS Foundation Trust, Birmingham, UK

Alex Wright [Chapters 37, 38]
Retired Consultant Diabetologist and Diabetic Eye Disease Specialist, University Hospitals Birmingham NHS Foundation Trust, Birmingham, UK

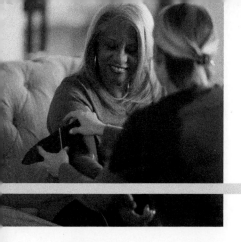

Acknowledgements

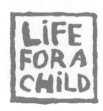

The Editor and authors wish to donate all Book royalties to the International Diabetes Federation Life for a Child https://www.idf.org/our-activities/humanitarian-action/life-for-a-child.html.

We wish to thank Richard Smith, Academic Learning Technologist, BCU, who gave enormous help with the illustrations.

Introduction

Part 1

Chapters

1 Diabetes prevention

Figure 1.1 Graph to show rising HbA1c levels and diagnosis of type 2 diabetes.

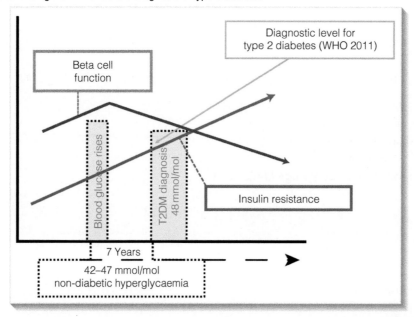

Diagnostic level for
type 2 diabetes (WHO 2011)

Beta cell
function

Blood glucose rises

T2DM diagnosis
48 mmol/mol

Insulin resistance

7 Years

42–47 mmol/mol
non-diabetic hyperglycaemia

Figure 1.3 One Less Challenge. *Source:* Africa Studio/Adobe Stock.

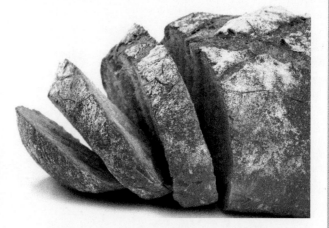

Figure 1.2 HbA1c.

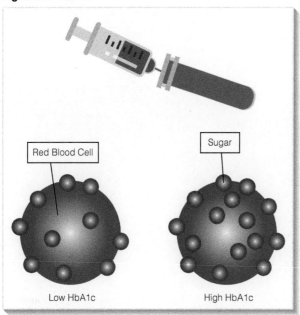

Red Blood Cell

Sugar

Low HbA1c

High HbA1c

Figure 1.4 Signs and symptoms of metabolic syndrome.

Lethargy

Tiredness

Difficulty concentrating

Weight gain (especially around the middle)

Hypertension

Hyperlipaemia

Hyperglycaemia

Diabetes Care at a Glance, First Edition. Edited by Anne Phillips.
© 2023 John Wiley & Sons Ltd. Published 2023 by John Wiley & Sons Ltd.

This chapter is to help you understand what diabetes prevention involves and how you can help people at risk of type 2 diabetes to reduce their risk. A record number of people across the UK and worldwide are living with type 2 diabetes, and this figure has more than doubled since 1996. The International Diabetes Federation (IDF 2021) reported that 537 million people are known to have diabetes worldwide, with predictions that this will rise to 783 million by 2045.

Type 2 diabetes is largely preventable, and the World Health Organization (WHO 2019) has recognized that diabetes predominantly affects people who are most vulnerable, with three in four adults with diabetes aged 20–79 living in low- and middle-income countries. Diabetes costs the worldwide health-care system at least £720 billion, a rise of 316% in total health expenditure since 2006.

Every two minutes someone discovers they have type 2 diabetes, a serious health condition that can cause long-term health problems. Type 2 diabetes causes about 90% of all types of diabetes worldwide. Intervention to prevent type 2 diabetes and target those most at risk of non-diabetic hyperglycaemia should be timely and outcomes can be favourable with early intervention and referral for people this affects.

Diabetes prevention programmes are becoming increasingly available worldwide. The programme in the UK is organized by NHS England, Public Health England and Diabetes UK and delivers a behavioural platform to support people in reducing their risk of developing type 2 diabetes, or in reversing the diagnosis if newly diagnosed. This programme is provided nationwide, and people can be referred via their GP practice or secondary care. The programme is delivered by different providers in primary care networks (**PCNs**) and involves a group class, a health coach and/or access to a personalized app to help motivate the patient to lose weight and be more physically active.

People are at risk when the level of HbA1c (an average of the last six to eight weeks of blood glucose levels) is raised (World Health Organization 2011). The diagnostic level of HbA1c for type 2 diabetes is 48 mmol/mol. Non-diabetic hyperglycaemia is diagnosed at 42–77 mmol/mol and this places people 'at risk' for type 2 diabetes (Figure 1.1). The interval from the onset of rising HbA1c levels to the diagnosis of type 2 diabetes is on average seven years; this period is a window of opportunity that allows the detection of non-diabetic hyperglycaemia and appropriate prevention strategies to be offered. Measurement of HbA1c is usually undertaken during a routine health review in general practice but might also take place during a preoperative screening or as part of an inpatient biochemistry profile.

HbA1c reflects the amount of glucose that binds to red blood cells (**RBCs**) when they are manufactured in the bone marrow. The blood glucose level at the time the RBCs are produced is the amount that binds to those RBCs for their lifespan, on average 12 weeks (Figure 1.2). Thus an HbA1c measurement comprises some older RBCs, some newer ones and some middle-aged ones, so that the HbA1c value is considered the average of all these RBCs, thus allowing six to eight weeks of glucose control.

The NHS National Diabetes Prevention Programme (Diabetes 2022) in the UK focuses on three main goals of behavioural intervention: (i) weight loss, (ii) achievement of individualized dietary recommendations, and (iii) achievement of recommended individualized physical activity recommendations. Person-centred goal setting with each individual is essential to engage people with their programme and to support each individual in achieving their personal goals in diabetes prevention and health gain. One approach for weight loss is to recommend 'one less' as this can be easily understood and can be meaningful for people to engage with. For example, one less slice of bread is equivalent to a saving of 32 kcal, and over seven days this amounts to 224 kcal less consumed (Figure 1.3). This can be adapted into people's daily routines and built upon by individuals as they achieve some weight reduction.

Screening people for diabetes can help to find people at high risk. Health professionals have a number of strategies to try to prevent type 2 diabetes and engage people in their own personal health. The Diabetes UK three-minute 'at risk' assessment is a good approach to use (https://riskscore.diabetes.org.uk/start) as this is individualized and offers support for people in their own homes (Figure 1.4).

References

Diabetes UK (2022). NHS Diabetes Prevention Programme. www.diabetes.org.uk/professionals/resources/shared-practice/nhs-diabetes-prevention-programme (accessed 1 April 2022).

International Diabetes Federation (2021). *IDF Diabetes Atlas*, 10e. https://diabetesatlas.org (accessed 1 April 2022).

World Health Organization (2011). *Use of glycated haemoglobin (HbA1c) in the diagnosis of diabetes mellitus. Abbreviated report of a WHO consultation*. WHO/NMH/CHP/ CPM/11.1. Geneva: World Health Organization https://apps.who.int/iris/handle/10665/70523 (accessed 1 April 2022).

World Health Organization (2019). Diabetes. www.who.int/news-room/fact-sheets/detail/diabetes (accessed 1 April 2022).

2 Diagnosis of type 1 diabetes

Figure 2.1 Lack of insulin causing type 1 diabetes.

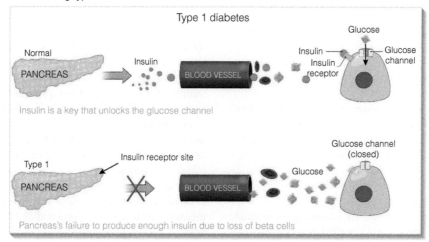

Figure 2.2 Symptoms of diabetes.

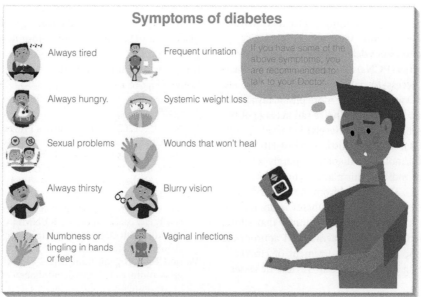

Figure 2.3 Diabetes UK 4Ts campaign.

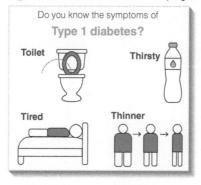

Diabetes Care at a Glance, First Edition. Edited by Anne Phillips.
© 2023 John Wiley & Sons Ltd. Published 2023 by John Wiley & Sons Ltd.

Type 1 diabetes is an autoimmune disease that develops when the body attacks and destroys approximately 80–90% of the beta cells in the pancreas that produce insulin. As a result of no longer producing insulin, most people with type 1 diabetes must inject insulin (see Chapter 16) every day throughout their lives or wear a small pump that continuously infuses insulin (see Chapter 17). A tiny proportion of people have new beta cells transplanted so they no longer require daily insulin replacement. Why the body attacks its beta cells is not fully understood, but genetics and environmental factors increase the risks.

The absence of insulin production in the pancreas (Figure 2.1) means that glucose cannot be absorbed from the bloodstream and the blood glucose level rises above the normal range (note that the term 'blood glucose' is commonly used to refer to plasma glucose levels). In people without type 1 diabetes, normal fasting blood glucose levels range between 4.0 and 5.4 mmol/l and can rise up to 7.8 mmol/l two hours after eating. Someone with newly diagnosed type 1 diabetes may present with high blood glucose levels (hyperglycaemia) ranging from 8 to 30 mmol/l or more.

The common signs and symptoms of type 1 diabetes are caused by a lack of insulin and the resulting high glucose levels (Figure 2.2). These include increased frequency of urination and passing large amounts of urine (polyuria). The body excretes glucose in the urine when blood glucose levels are above 9 or 10 mmol/l. Increased thirst develops (polydipsia) as the body seeks to replace the fluid lost due to increased urination. People with new onset of undiagnosed type 1 diabetes may often present with increased appetite (polyphagia) and fatigue. Glucose provides fuel to cells throughout the body, so without insulin glucose remains in the bloodstream and the cells are starved of the fuel they need to function properly. Weight loss is likely to occur as the body breaks down fat to use as an alternative fuel source. This leads to a build-up of ketone bodies in the bloodstream. Fruity-smelling breath is a sign of high blood ketones. High levels of ketones in the blood can result in metabolic acidosis and diabetic ketoacidosis (DKA), a life-threatening emergency (see Chapter 24).

Healthcare professionals should be familiar with the classic signs and symptoms of type 1 diabetes such as polyuria, polydipsia, polyphagia, fatigue, weight loss, fruity-smelling breath and blurred vision, which may develop over a short time period. Clinicians who recognize these should take urgent action to diagnose and manage type 1 diabetes.

Diagnosing type 1 diabetes

Unavoidable deaths due to missed diagnosis of type 1 diabetes still occur. Within primary care settings, testing a fingerstick blood sample and/or urine for glucose and ketones can quickly identify high glucose levels.

Referrals to hospital enable further blood tests to confirm the diagnosis. Anti-islet cell antibodies are likely to be present in most people with newly diagnosed type 1 diabetes and may confirm the diagnosis. Low C-peptide levels may also indicate a lack of insulin production.

Type 1 diabetes can be diagnosed in people of any age. Approximately 400 000 people, including 30 000 children, live with type 1 diabetes in the UK (National Institute for Health and Care Excellence 2022a,b). Diabetes UK launched their 4Ts campaign (Figure 2.3) to promote the four main symptoms of type 1 diabetes as so many late diagnoses were occurring where symptoms had been missed or overlooked. This campaign is nationally advertised to try to inform the public to seek help if they or a family member is experiencing any of these symptoms.

Support post diagnosis to help people adjust and learn how to live with type 1 diabetes is essential. Learning to monitor blood glucose and inject insulin and how to balance insulin dose requirements with food and physical activity does take time and adjustment to gain self-confidence while living with type 1 diabetes.

Honeymoon period

Some people with newly diagnosed type 1 diabetes may experience a short remission phase, also known as the honeymoon period, when they require very little insulin to normalize their glucose levels. This occurs because the remaining pancreatic beta cells (approximately 10–20%) continue to produce insulin after initial high glucose values have fallen after starting insulin therapy.

Skills for self-managing type 1 diabetes

To self-manage type 1 diabetes, people must invest time to monitor their glucose levels and adjust the amount of insulin they inject or infuse according to their diet (specifically carbohydrates), activity levels, stress and a number of other factors. Structured education courses such as DAFNE and BERTIE provide people with opportunities to learn self-management skills and also meet other people living with type 1 diabetes. Ideally, people would be invited to attend a course within 6–12 months of being diagnosed with type 1 diabetes. However, people may still benefit from attending many years after their diagnosis (see Chapter 8).

References

National Institute for Health and Care Excellence (2022a). Type 1 Diabetes in Adults: Diagnosis and Management. NICE Guideline NG17. Available at www.nice.org.uk/guidance/ng17

National Institute for Health and Care Excellence (2022b). Diabetes (Type 1 and Type 2) in Children and Young People: Diagnosis and Management. NICE Guideline NG18. Available at www.nice.org.uk/guidance/ng18.

3 Diagnosis of type 2 diabetes

Figure 3.1 How insulin resistance occurs.

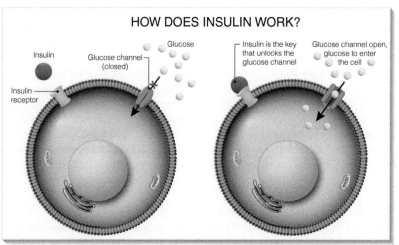

Figure 3.2 Metabolic syndrome.

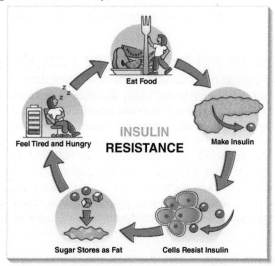

Figure 3.4 Diagnosis of type 2 diabetes.

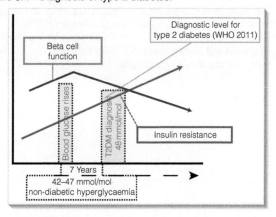

Figure 3.3 Signs and symptoms of metabolic syndrome.

- Lethargy
- Tiredness
- Difficulty concentrating
- Weight gain (especially around the middle)
- Hypertension
- Hyperlipaemia
- Hyperglycaemia

Figure 3.5 HbA1c.

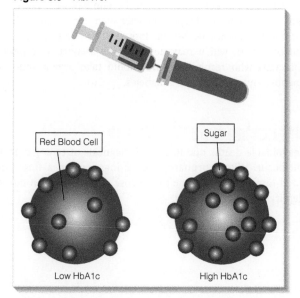

Diabetes Care at a Glance, First Edition. Edited by Anne Phillips.
© 2023 John Wiley & Sons Ltd. Published 2023 by John Wiley & Sons Ltd.

Every year World Diabetes Day takes place globally on 14 November, but despite this campaign to raise awareness type 2 diabetes remains inadequately diagnosed. Early diagnosis of type 2 diabetes is vital to prevent further illness and the subsequent complications. Type 2 diabetes is a major public health concern because of its increasing incidence and prevalence worldwide, and the increased risk and health concerns associated with the diagnosis of diabetes.

Among ethnic community minorities, the prevalence of type 2 diabetes is alarmingly higher than in White populations, and people of South Asian ancestry, for example, present approximately 10 years earlier than White people, with a significant proportion of cases being diagnosed before the age of 40 years (Goff 2019). Type 2 diabetes can also present as 'lean type 2' in individuals with lower body mass index (BMI) and normal weight particularly (Goff 2019).

Insulin resistance often precedes the diagnosis of type 2 diabetes. Insulin resistance manifests when the insulin receptors on muscle cell membranes (Figure 3.1) do not respond to the insulin produced and cannot use glucose in the blood for energy, so glucose is stored as fat. Insulin resistance is initially symptomless but progresses as blood glucose levels rise. When this occurs, other symptoms such as the metabolic syndrome presents, with high blood pressure (hypertension), elevated cholesterol levels (hyperlipaemia) and elevated glucose levels (hyperglycaemia) (Figure 3.2).

Type 2 diabetes and its associated comorbidities are growing more prevalent. Cardiovascular disease remains the largest cause of mortality and morbidity in people with type 2 diabetes (Seidu et al. 2022). To identify type 2 diabetes promptly, a good knowledge of the risk factors and of the presenting symptoms (or lack of them) is important. Risk factors for developing type 2 diabetes are shown in Figure 3.3. The diagnosis of type 2 diabetes is usually made in adulthood, although increasing numbers of children and young people aged under 18 years are being diagnosed, usually in association with obesity and other risk factors.

The renal threshold describes the blood glucose level at which the kidneys filter glucose into the urine to create glucosuria. This varies from person to person and some people, for example pregnant women and older people, can have lower renal thresholds so present with glucosuria without diabetes. Diabetes cannot be diagnosed via urinalysis alone and this needs to be followed up with HbA1c measurement in accordance with World Health Organization (WHO 2011) guidance. It is important to remember that it is relatively rare for glucose to be present in urine, so this needs further investigation.

In someone with symptoms (Figure 3.4), an HbA1c of 48 mmol/mol or more on a single occasion confirms the diagnosis of type 2 diabetes (NICE 2015). In the absence of symptoms, the HbA1c should be repeated within two weeks to clarify the diagnosis (WHO 2011). HbA1c is measured by laboratory testing of venous blood using a tube containing ethylenediaminetetraacetic acid (**EDTA**) (Figure 3.5). It is important to ensure a correct diagnosis and to undertake this in a timely manner as type 2 diabetes can lead to many preventable cardiovascular, neuropathic and psychological complications if diagnosed late. Many people are diagnosed opportunistically during general practice health reviews and, as discussed in the previous chapter, early diagnosis and screening is a pivotal opportunity to begin diabetes prevention strategies to help people into remission.

Type 2 diabetes is a progressive condition that will require increasing medication and education to help individuals cope with their condition. Treatment escalation using individualized and person-centred approaches is essential to help people learn about and self-manage their type 2 diabetes well.

If type 2 diabetes is diagnosed later when a complication arises, for example following a myocardial infarction (heart attack) or on presentation of a foot ulcer, this represents a missed opportunity for earlier diagnosis and can lead to patient distress and inadvertent blaming of the individual for the diabetes. Sadly, there are still many late diagnoses and 50% of people still present at diagnosis with established complications of diabetes (Seidu et al. 2022).

References

Goff, L.M. (2019). Ethnicity and type 2 diabetes in the UK. *Diabet. Med.* 36 (8): 927–938. https://doi.org/10.1111/dme.13895.

National Institute for Health and Care Excellence (2015). Type 2 Diabetes in Adults: Management. NICE Guideline NG28. www.nice.org.uk/guidance/ng28.

Seidu, S., Cos, X., Brunton, S. et al. (2022). 2022 Update to the position statement by Primary Care Diabetes Europe: a disease state approach to the pharmacological management of type 2 diabetes in primary care. *Prim. Care Diabetes* 16: 223–244.

World Health Organization (2011). *Use of glycated haemoglobin (HbA1c) in the diagnosis of diabetes mellitus. Abbreviated report of a WHO consultation.* WHO/NMH/CHP/ CPM/11.1. Geneva: World Health Organization https://apps.who.int/iris/handle/10665/70523.

4 Consultation approaches and language matters

Figure 4.1 NHS England (2018) *Language Matters*. *Source:* NHS England 2018.

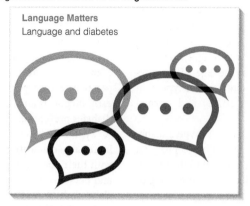

Figure 4.2 Modelling language from *Language Matters*.

Modelling language

The *Language Matters* guidance from NHS England (2018) provides some suggested words and phrases that you can model. These are guides that can be adapted to your own preferences, keeping true to the communication principles. The table below provides some practical examples to consider.

Avoid	Consider replacing with an alternative, such as	Communication style
"Before you come to see me, I want you take 4 blood tests a day for 3 days, so I can check what's going wrong"	"It may be helpful to do some more blood glucose monitoring, so we can better see the patterns. In an ideal world, as many as 4 a day for 3 days would be great, but I realise that's challenging! What feels manageable to you?"	Demanding → collaborative
"Your HbA$_{1c}$ is too high"	"Your HbA$_{1c}$ this time is higher than recommended"	Judgemental → fact-based
"It's being so overweight that is causing you to have all these problems"	"There are many reasons why we eat. Would you like to talk about them?"	Shaming → curious
"The diabetics/patients I support tend to find *xyz* helpful"	"The people with diabetes I support tend to find *xyz* helpful"	Condition-first language → person-first language
"Why were you so high here?" (when looking at a blood glucose monitoring diary)	"I can see your blood glucose levels were higher here. Can you recall what was going on that day?"	Deamanding → explorative
"You're not compliant"	"Diabetes can be difficult to manage every day. What gets in the way for you?"	Labelling → explorative
You don't acknowledge that appointments are running late when you greet the person.	"I'm seeing you later than your appointment time and I appreciate you waiting"	Unboundaried → respectful of boundaries (which fosters trust)
"You're in denial"	"Many people I support find it difficult to come to terms with their diabetes. This is natural and the process often takes time"	Stigmatising → empathic

Diabetes Care at a Glance, First Edition. Edited by Anne Phillips.
© 2023 John Wiley & Sons Ltd. Published 2023 by John Wiley & Sons Ltd.

The choice of words healthcare professionals use can and does have a profound impact on the recipient. The context of the conversation holds meaning and as such can be potentially helpful or harmful. Where the conversation takes place and if this is linked to a diagnosis of diabetes will be remembered for a long time. As Rudyard Kipling wrote 'Words are, after all, the most powerful drug used by mankind'. Using appropriate language and ensuring people understand what is being said and why costs nothing. Communication is a skill and as health professionals it is essential our skills are worked upon so words can be used appropriately without causing lasting harm.

NHS England (2018) has published guidance called *Language Matters: Language and Diabetes*. This offers the wide-ranging thoughts and considerations of key stakeholders, including people with diabetes, about how consultation conversations, wherever these take place, can be improved by use of appropriate language (Figure 4.1). It is important to acknowledge that despite the ever-increasing options in treatment, education approaches and self-management opportunities, the proportion of people with diabetes who can maintain a good HbA1c and gain healthy outcomes remains low (Bateman 2021). The diagnosis of diabetes provides a valuable opportunity to open a window of conversations to build a partnership with people with diabetes. Words are powerful and if delivered in a rushed insensitive manner, the context will be lost and harm can be caused. Language matters and it is worth taking time to prepare for conversations and reflect on the words you plan to use. For example, quotes from the research that went into preparing *Language Matters* (Figure 4.1) demonstrate the impact of conversations for people with diabetes. Figure 4.2 demonstrates some approaches advocated by *Language Matters* that should be adopted into your practice.

As Bateman (2021) recognized, words do more than reflect life, they create experience and language reflects and shapes people's thoughts, reactions and feelings. Words can reinforce beliefs or labels. Words can impact self-confidence and motivation. Words can influence choice and impact on physical and emotional well-being. Words can affect trust and need to be used to promote support, collaboration and empathy. Judgement, stigmatization and blame must be avoided in all conversations and must be recognized in others to allow challenge of the approaches used. Labelling must also be avoided, so do not use terms like 'diabetic' or 'diabetics' but replace with 'person with diabetes' or 'patient with diabetes'. This represents a person-centred approach and places the person first as an individual before their condition.

Making every contact count (Health Education England 2022) is an essential part of your practice: offer everyone you speak to some encouragement about an aspect of their health, impart a sense of the importance of diabetes while at the same time conveying a sense of hope and optimism that you are here to help. Being person-centred and offering individualized approaches helps people recognize they matter as an individual. Their experience of diabetes and their understanding of their health is ultimately what will guide their decision-making (Figure 4.2). Being there to offer support and understanding in a partnership approach encourages people to feel understood and cared for. Taking a few extra minutes to ensure you are talking with the individual and not over them is best practice. Talking about people in their hearing is alienating and creates barriers. Even if you meet a person with diabetes on one occasion only during their care, you can make so much difference. Your approach and the words you use in that interaction can make that contact count in a positive way. Including people in decisions about them and their diabetes is vital and respects their choices. This reflects the Department of Health (2012) declaration 'No decision about me, without me' and will help healthcare professionals display inclusion and promotion of positive conversations using language that is meaningful and helpful.

References

Bateman, J. (2021). How to find the ideal words in consultations. *Diabet. Prim. Care* 23: 71.

Department of Health (2012). Liberating the NHS: No Decision About Me, Without Me. https://assets.publishing.service.gov.uk/government/uploads/system/uploads/attachment_data/file/216980/Liberating-the-NHS-No-decision-about-me-without-me-Government-response.pdf.

Health Education England (2022). Making every contact count. www.makingeverycontactcount.co.uk.

NHS England (2018). Language Matters: Language and Diabetes. http://bit.ly/3t0UQXg.

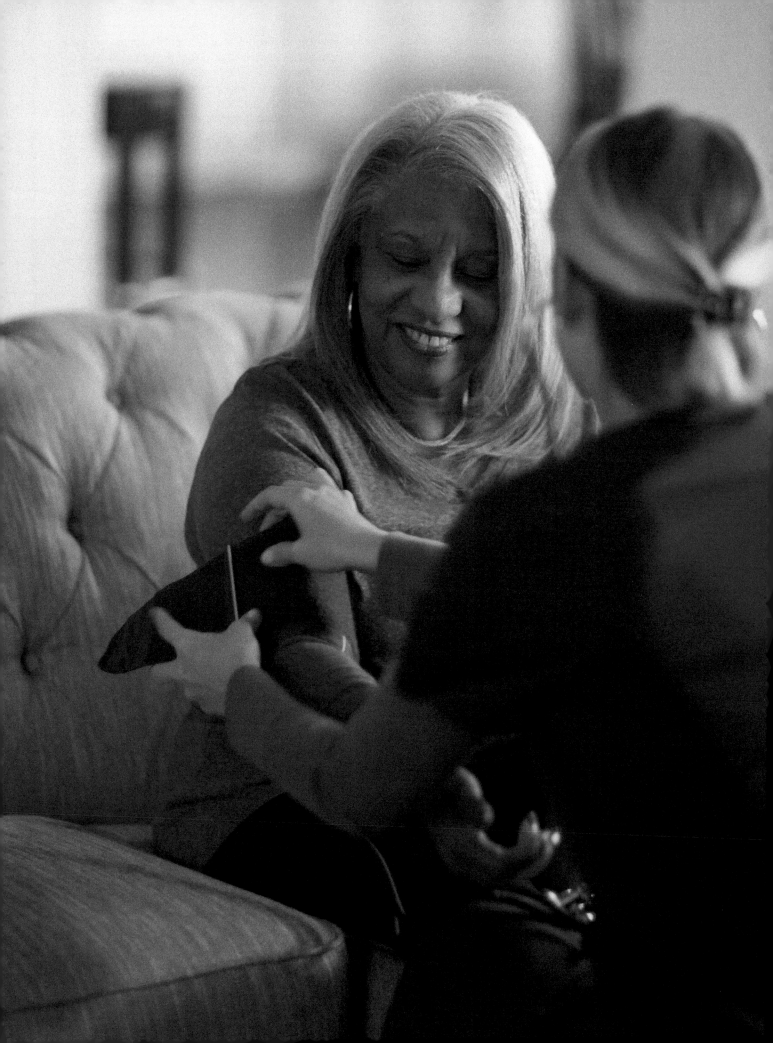

Principles of diabetes care

Part 2

Chapters

5 Promotion of healthy eating

Figure 5.1 The eat well plate.

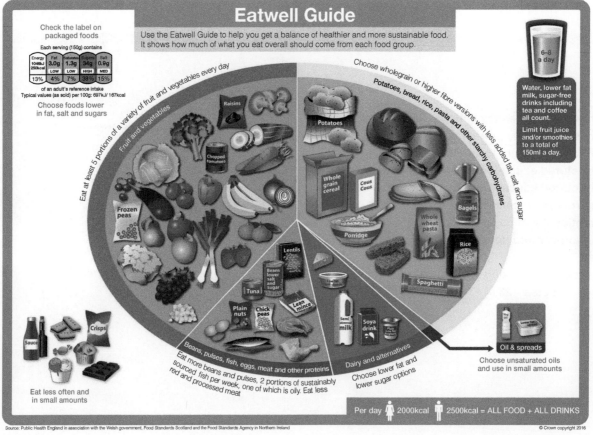

The Eatwell Guide (Figure 5.1) shows the proportions of the main food groups that form a healthy balanced diet for the general population and includes the following sections (Figure 5.2).

The yellow section

Carbohydrate is the body's main energy source. Starch is broken down to produce glucose which is used by the body for energy.

Diabetes mellitus is a complex condition that results from a combination of genetic predisposition, environmental factors and metabolic changes. It is these metabolic changes that alter glucose regulation. All dietary carbohydrate affects postprandial glucose levels. Manipulating dietary intake while simultaneously balancing nutritional quality is a key strategy in supporting glycaemic control. The misuse of glucose as the main energy substrate leads to hyperglycaemia.

For those with diabetes, carbohydrate intake can be manipulated in terms of total daily intake, meal distribution and portion size to support glycaemic control and weight management. Carbohydrate awareness, knowledge of reading food labels and the use of visual aids such as food models, apps and books showing carbohydrate portion sizes are useful educational resources

that support self-management. High-fibre, low glycaemic index foods can be useful as they slow digestive transit time and promote satiety, supporting portion management.

The green section

Fruit and vegetables contain high levels of micronutrients, including vitamins, minerals and antioxidants, that are essential to the multitude of biochemical processes carried out by the body. Furthermore, fruit and vegetables are a good source of dietary fibre, which has positive health benefits for the gut, and are also generally low in calories. Current guidance for the UK is to eat at least five portions daily and can be eaten in a variety of forms (fresh, dried, frozen and tinned).

The blue section

Milk, cheese, yoghurts and calcium-fortified alternatives are the body's main source of calcium, necessary for growth, development and healthy bones and teeth. Dairy sources are also a good source of protein (pink section). It is important to be aware that milk, cheese, cream and milk-based sauces can have a high saturated fat content, so looking for products with a reduced fat content

Diabetes Care at a Glance, First Edition. Edited by Anne Phillips.
© 2023 John Wiley & Sons Ltd. Published 2023 by John Wiley & Sons Ltd.

Figure 5.2 Principles of healthy eating.

- Choose low glycaemic index sources of carbohydrates whilst being very much aware of the portion sizes served and consumed (yellow section).
- Eat at least five portions of a variety of fruit and vegetables every day (green section).
- Have some dairy or dairy alternatives (such as soya drinks), choosing lower fat and lower sugar options (blue section).
- Eat some beans, pulses, fish, eggs, meat and other proteins, including two portions of fish every week, one of which should be oily (pink section).
- Choose unsaturated oils and spreads and eat in small amounts (purple section)
- Drink six to eight cups/glasses of fluid a day.
- If consuming foods and drinks high in fat, salt or sugar have these less often and in small amounts.

Figure 5.4 Visual guide to what a plate could look like.

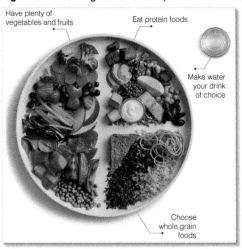

Have plenty of vegetables and fruits

Eat protein foods

Make water your drink of choice

Choose whole grain foods

Figure 5.3 What is a portion? *Source:* Daniel Thornberg / Adobe Stock; azure / Adobe Stock; pixelrobot / Adobe Stock; MAGINE / Adobe Stock; cherezoff / Adobe Stock ; Africa Studio / Adobe Stock; Željko Radojko / Adobe Stock.

Object	Hand symbol	Equivalent	Foods
		First 1 cup (baseball)	Rice, Pasta Fruit Veggies
		Palm 1/2 cup (tennis ball)	Medium fruit, Ice cream
		Palm 3 ounces (deck of cards)	Meat Fish Poultry
		Handful 1 ounce (1 large egg)	Nuts Raisins
		2 Handfuls 1 ounce (2 large eggs)	Chips Popcorn Pretzels
		Thumb 1 ounce (ping pong ball)	Peanut butter Hard cheese
		Thumb tip 1 teaspoon (marble)	Cooking oil Mayonnaise, Butter, Sugar

may be helpful. Yoghurts can have a high sugar content so look for products using a sweetener rather than sugar.

The pink section

Protein is available from both animal sources including meat, fish, eggs and dairy (milks, yoghurts and cheeses) and plant sources including nuts, seeds and pulses e.g. peas, beans, lentils and includes soybean curd (Tofu) as well as mycoproteins (Quorn) which can therefore count as part of the five a day regime (green section).

Protein sources contain iron and vitamin B_{12} (meat and fish) and essential fatty acids such as omega-3 (oily fish like mackerel, salmon and sardines). One portion of white fish and one portion of oily fish is recommended per week.

Recent research recommends a reduction in the consumption of red meat (beef, lamb, goat and pork) as this would be better for both our health and the environment.

The purple section

Dietary fats have important functions within the body. In addition, and like carbohydrate, fat also provides energy but is far denser (more calories in a smaller volume). The different types of fat have different effects on the body and especially on cholesterol levels.

- Essential fatty acids: these are not produced by the body and need to be consumed, for example omega-3 oils, found in the flesh of oily fish and skin of whitefish. They can also be found in some plant sources such as flaxseed, rapeseed and soya but are

present in much smaller amounts. Omega-3 oils are protective against heart disease.

- Saturated fats: These can increase the level of low-density lipoprotein (LDL) cholesterol and increase the risk of heart disease and other circulatory problems. They are found in animal fats and processed foods.

- Unsaturated fats: these are generally found in vegetable oils (e.g. olive, rapeseed and seed oils). They generally contain high-density lipoprotein (HDL) cholesterol, which can reduce harmful LDL cholesterol.

Salt

High levels of salt in the diet can increase blood pressure. Most of the salt we consume is in processed foods (ready meals and snack foods). It is recommended that we do not consume more than 6 g (one teaspoon) per day.

Portion sizes

Giving practical advice with respect to portion sizes is important and this can be undertaken by a visual guide to portion size for the different food groups (Figure 5.3) and a visual guide to what a meal could look like (Figure 5.4).

The annual diabetes review appointment provides the ideal opportunity to review an individual's dietary and lifestyle progress with regard to biochemical markers such as lipid levels and HbA1c, and to also monitor anthropometric markers such as weight and waist circumference.

6 Physical activity promotion

Figure 6.1 Different levels of exercise intensity and their effects on the body.

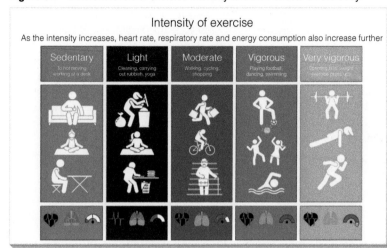

Figure 6.2 MET examples.

Sitting = 1 MET
Walking at 3 mph = 3–6 METs
Gardening = 3–6 METS
Leisure cycling <10 mph = 3–6 METS
Ballroom dancing = 3–6 METS
Low impact aerobics = 3–6 METS
High impact aerobics = ≥6 METs
Walking uphill carrying a 10kg load = ≥6 METS
Heavy digging = ≥6 METS
Cycling moderate effort >12 mph = ≥6 METS

Figure 6.3 Different examples of aerobic and anaerobic exercise.

Aerobic:
Swimming
Cycling
Walking
Rowing
Jogging for 10 minutes
Dancing

Anaerobic:
Weight-lifting
Pilates
Yoga
sprints

Figure 6.4 Glucose utilization during anaerobic and aerobic exercise and after rest.

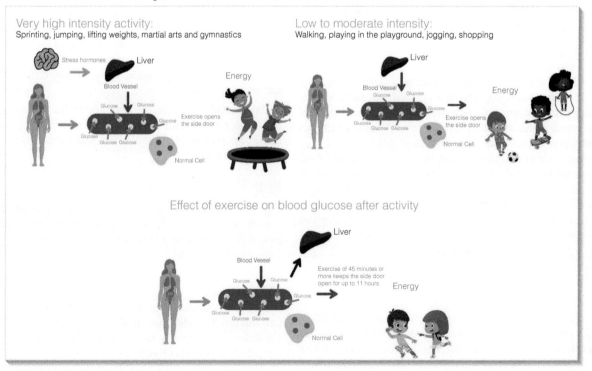

Diabetes Care at a Glance, First Edition. Edited by Anne Phillips.
© 2023 John Wiley & Sons Ltd. Published 2023 by John Wiley & Sons Ltd.

Engagement in and promotion of physical activity are central factors in diabetes care. Type 1 diabetes is a challenging condition to manage for a variety of physiological and behavioural reasons. Regular exercise is important, but management of different forms of physical activity can be particularly difficult for both the individual with type 1 diabetes and the health professional. Several barriers can exist for people with diabetes, including fear of hypoglycaemia, loss of glycaemic control and inadequate knowledge about exercise management.

Physical activity, along with nutritional advice, are essential factors in the prevention and control of type 2 diabetes since their effects influence blood pressure, glycaemia and lipidaemia. Evidence has shown that aerobic, resistance or combined exercise programmes are some of the best types of non-pharmacological treatments for controlling type 2 diabetes and managing weight (Figure 6.1).

Physical activity can be described as any movement of skeletal muscles that results in energy expenditure. Examples include household activities like gardening, walking a dog, carrying heavy loads and doing the weekly shopping. Increasing physical activity is beneficial and can be measured in METS. A MET is quantified by determining the ratio of an individual's metabolic rate when undertaking a specific activity to their basal metabolic rate when resting. Examples of MET expenditure are shown in Figure 6.2.

In order to help people become more active for a healthier world, the World Health Organization (2018) published its Global Action Plan on Physical Activity 2018–2030. This report showed that worldwide one in four adults and three in four young people (13–19 years) do not meet the global recommendations for physical activity. As countries develop economically, levels of inactivity increase due to changing patterns of transport and increased use of technology. Physical activity is also influenced by cultural values, for example girls, women, older adults and economically disadvantaged communities have less access to and fewer opportunities for safe, affordable and appropriate programmes and safe places in which to be physically active.

Engagement in regular physical activity provides a range of physical and mental health benefits, and increasing the type and intensity of the exercise gradually can motivate people to achieve more and increase their confidence and self-esteem. The recommendations for type 2 diabetes are 30 minutes every day, without stopping if possible; if this is not achievable immediately, the individual should try for three 10-minute stints to build up stamina and success. Moderate and vigorous activity can be differentiated by the 'talk test': being able to talk but not sing indicates moderate physical activity; having difficulty talking without pausing is a sign of vigorous physical activity. This is a good way to explain the concept to people with diabetes.

In type 1 diabetes, aerobic and anaerobic exercise require different management approaches. Aerobic exercise involves endurance-type exercises that require oxygen to generate energy. Anaerobic exercise involves short, intense bursts of physical activity. Examples of both types are shown in Figure 6.3.

The *UK Chief Medical Officers' Physical Activity Guidelines* (Department of Social Care 2019) recommend that adults engage in 150–300 minutes of moderate aerobic activity or 75–150 minutes of vigorous intense aerobic activity every week. Increasing the amount of exercise will provide greater health benefits. Aerobic exercises increase a person's heart rate and breathing rate in order to increase oxygen uptake for the body's muscle function. Aerobic exercise can increase stamina, lower blood pressure, increase high-density lipoprotein (HDL) cholesterol, and improve mood and sleep. Reduction of insulin and eating carbohydrates before exercise can help maintain glucose levels and avoid hypoglycaemia after exercise. Diligence in testing glucose levels before, during and after aerobic exercise can help individuals learn how to self-manage engagement in different types of activities and also to enjoy them more. This approach can reduce delayed hypoglycaemia, which can occur many hours after exercise. See Figure 6.4 for the effects of different forms of exercise on glucose metabolism.

Anaerobic exercise is recommended on at least two days per week. It is important to engage in a warm-up and cool-down activity when engaging in anaerobic activity as this can reduce the lactic acid released during this type of activity. The production of lactic acid indicates that carbohydrate or glucose is not being used for fuel, and the build-up of lactic acid can cause muscle cramps.

Drinking water during all forms of exercise helps to reduce lactic acid, maintains hydration and increases pleasure from the activity also.

References

Department of Social Care (2019). UK Chief Medical Officers' Physical Activity Guidelines https://assets.publishing.service.gov.uk/government/uploads/system/uploads/attachment_data/file/832868/uk-chief-medical-officers-physical-activity-guidelines.pdf.

World Health Organization (2018). *Global Action Plan on Physical Activity 2018–2030. More Active People for a Healthier World.* Geneva: World Health Organization https://apps.who.int/iris/bitstream/handle/10665/272722/9789241514187-eng.pdf.

7 Promoting weight loss

Figure 7.1 Classification of obesity in adults based on BMI (kg/m²).

Classification of obesity in adults based on BMI (kg/m²)	
Underweight	≤18.5
Healthy/normal weight	18.5–24.9
Overweight (pre obese)	25–29.9
Moderate obesity (class 1)	30–34.9
Severe obesity (class 2)	35–39.9
Morbid obesity (class 3)	≥ 40

Figure 7.2 Waist circumference thresholds as a measure of obesity.

Waist circumference thresholds as a measure of obesity		
	Waist circumference in cm.	
	European populations	South Asian, Chinese and Japanese populations
Men	≥94	≥90
Women	≥80	≥80

Figure 7.3 Relative risk for obese people developing associated diseases.

Relative risk for obese people developing associated diseases		
Disease	**Women**	**Men**
Type 2 diabetes	12.7	5.2
Hypertension	4.2	2.6
Myocardial infarction	3.2	1.5
Colon cancer	2.7	3.0
Angina	1.8	1.8
Gallbladder diseases	1.8	1.8
Ovarian cancer	1.7	-
Osteoarthritis	1.4	1.9
Stroke	1.3	1.3

Figure 7.4 The benefits of a 10% weight loss (10-kg weight loss based on a body weight of 100 kg).

The benefits of a 10% weight loss. A 10 kg weight loss based on a body weight of 100 kg	
Mortality	>20% fall in total mortality
	>30% fall in diabetes-related deaths
	>40% fall in obesity-related cancer deaths
Blood pressure	A fall of 10 mmHg systolic
	A fall of 20 mmHg diastolic
Diabetes	A 50% fall in the risk of developing type 2 diabetes
	A fall of 50% in fasting glucose
	A 15% decrease in HbA1c
Lipids	A fall of 10% total cholesterol
	A fall of 15% in LDL (low-density lipoprotein)
	A fall of 30% triglycerides
	An increase of 8% in HDL (high-density lipoprotein)

Diabetes Care at a Glance, First Edition. Edited by Anne Phillips.
© 2023 John Wiley & Sons Ltd. Published 2023 by John Wiley & Sons Ltd.

Obesity is a well-known risk factor for the development of type 2 diabetes. It is estimated that 60–90% of type 2 diabetes is directly related to obesity. Increasing weight, particularly central obesity as indicated by an increased girth measurement, leads to insulin resistance. In an attempt to maintain glucose homeostasis, the beta cells of the pancreas produce increasing amounts of insulin (hyperinsulinaemia), which leads to deterioration and possible failure of beta-cell function.

Obesity is by far the greatest risk factor in the development of type 2 diabetes, and in turn is responsible for the increasing global prevalence of diabetes (International Diabetes Federation 2022). The coexistence of obesity and diabetes has led to a new concept of 'diabesity', and this has implications for treatment. Obesity is caused by an excess of energy intake over and above an individual's daily energy requirement, resulting in that energy being stored. Energy is stored as fat and may be deposited subcutaneously and viscerally.

Obesity can be determined by calculating a person's body mass index (BMI), which is the ratio of weight in kilograms to height in metres squared. The BMI value is then used to classify obesity based on the World Health Organization (WHO) guidelines (2022) (Figure 7.1). Unfortunately, BMI does not take into consideration a person's body composition, i.e. the ratio of visceral and subcutaneous fat and muscle. This is important when assessing obesity. People with a high muscle mass, such as sportsmen especially rugby players, may be seen as being obese. The use of waist circumference in conjunction with BMI can give a clearer picture of a person's risk of obesity (Figure 7.2).

With increasing body weight there is an increasing risk of ill health, and the National Audit Office has examined the relative risks of developing other diseases for people who are obese (Figure 7.3). The report found that obese women were three times more likely to have a cardiovascular event compared with those who were not obese, while men were 1.5 times more likely. It is possible therefore that people newly diagnosed with type 2 diabetes are likely to have other comorbidities due to the underlying presence of obesity (Figure 7.3).

Adipose tissue is not simply a store for excess energy intake, but is biochemically active. The adipocytes (fat cells) are involved with the production and secretion of numerous enzymes, growth factors, cytokines and hormones that are involved in overall energy homeostasis. Unfortunately, as the level of obesity increases, the dysfunction of the adipocytes increases, promoting further weight gain and leading to obesity.

The evidence supporting the benefits of weight loss is clear and well documented for the clinician (Figure 7.4). However, from an individual's perspective, achieving any weight loss can be overwhelming, especially with previous failed attempts. Therefore, it is important for all health professionals to assess the patient's willingness, confidence and motivation to address weight loss, and then support the individual to agree lifestyle (diet and physical activity) change using SMART (Specific, Measurable, Achievable, Relevant to the goal of treatment and Time specific) targets. An appreciation for the transtheoretical approach to behaviour change will allow an appreciation of the cycle for change in behaviour planning taking action but being ready for relapse and moving on again.

Achieving long-term weight loss is not straightforward. Dietary behaviours are formed during childhood and are then shaped and developed by a multitude of experiences as the individual moves through adolescence into adult life. Therefore, food choices are complex and unique. As such, there is no panacea to losing weight.

There is a variety of approaches to weight loss but ultimately the aim is to address energy balance. The evidence-based nutrition guidelines for the prevention and management of diabetes (Diabetes UK 2018) place the emphasis on weight management. However, the guidelines also acknowledge that there is a variety of approaches available to tackle weight loss. There is uncertainty regarding which dietary intervention is the most successful so in practice it is important to work with patients, ensuring their safety and working in line with national guidance.

The role of the dietitian is to use specialist knowledge to translate complex nutritional information into practical dietary advice to support people in making appropriate food choices and to help achieve their aims through weight loss and, more importantly, weight maintenance. This strategy will also improve glycaemic control, long-term health and quality of life.

One of the benefits of physical activity is that it has an independent effect on glycaemic control. However, when used as the sole approach for weight loss it is not so effective. Using dietary changes in conjunction with physical activity will result in greater weight loss than diet or physical activity alone.

The adjustment of medications, especially insulin, for patients with type 2 diabetes who are increasing their physical activity and actively losing weight is very important for maintaining their safety and preventing the risk of hypoglycaemia. As diabetes evolves over time, beta-cell function also declines. When considering possible treatment options for patients who present with deterioration in long-term glycaemic control (HbA1c), it is important that health professionals remember that there is a greater variety of medications available for initial treatment to improve glycaemic control and minimize weight gain.

The annual review presents an ideal opportunity for discussing and promoting weight management while considering the patient's preferences and taking a collaborative approach to care planning, which in turn maximizes a patient-centred approach (see Chapter 29).

References

Diabetes UK (2018). Evidence-Based Nutrition Guidelines for the Prevention and Management of Diabetes. www.diabetes.org.uk/professionals/position-statements-reports/food-nutrition-lifestyle/evidence-based-nutrition-guidelines-for-the-prevention-and-management-of-diabetes.
International Diabetes Federation (2022). *IDF Diabetes Atlas*, 10e. https://diabetesatlas.org.
World Health Organization (2022). Obesity and overweight. https://www.who.int/news-room/fact-sheets/detail/obesity-and-overweight.

8 Structured education in type 1 diabetes

Figure 8.1 Example of type 1 diabetes structured education content. *Source:* Kiddell et al. (2019).

Box 1. STEP lesson plans.

Lesson plan 1 (delivered by DSN)
- What is type 1 diabetes?
- Fears and anxieties about diagnosis
- Blood glucose (BG) monitoring and targets
- Insulin
- Role of food
- Recognition and treatment of hypoglycaemia
- If applicable: driving, avoiding pregnancy at the moment, employment, statement of fitness to work

Lesson plan 2 (DSN)
- Recap what diabetes is
- Recap BG monitoring and targets
- Using Diasend
- Recap insulin
- Repeat prescriptions
- Recap role of food
- Recap recognition and treatment of hypos
- Future appointments
- If applicable: driving, smoking, avoiding pregnancy, employment

Lesson plan 3 (Dietitian)
- Introduce food groups
- Relationship between BG, carbohydrate (CHO) and insulin
- CHO counting introductions, reading labels, apps, reference tables, Carbs & Cals
- Food diary

Lesson plan 4 (DSN)
- Treatment of hypoglycaemia
- Effect of alcohol, exercise, hot weather, stress and lipohypertrophy/lipoatrophy on BG
- Hyperglycaemia
- Diabetic ketoacidosis

Lesson plan 5 (Dietitian)
- Review food diary
- Insulin-to-CHO ratio
- Insulin sensitivity factor
- Bolus advisor BG meter
- Food and BG diary

Lesson plan 6 (Dietitian)
- Review of food and BG diary
- Healthy living
- Alcohol

Lesson plan 7 (Consultant)
- Discuss existing health problems
- Screening: eyes, feet, weight
- BG targets and HbA1c
- Diasend upload
- If applicable: pregnancy planning, smoking

Lesson plan 8 (DSN)
- Reviewing results/Diasend
- Hypoglycaemia requiring third-party assistance
- Meter maintenance
- Future appointment
- If applicable: smart meter settings, holidays, driving, DVLA, effect of prolonged exercise on BG

Psychology-led group session
- Role of clinical psychology within diabetes
- Adjusting to life with diabetes
- Distress and coping
- Other areas of support

Consultant-led group session
- Staying healthy
- Screening
- Review home BG results
- Fears and concerns
- Future appointments

This chapter discusses the components of structured diabetes education for people living with type 1 diabetes and is based on guidance from the National Institute for Health and Care Excellence (2022). The first few months after diagnosis involves considerable adjustment, so information should be given from diagnosis. People with type 1 diabetes need to acquire a range of information and it is often said that education is the cornerstone of diabetes care. There are new skills and knowledge which are important in diabetes self-management. Managing their condition on a day-to-day basis is done with the support of their healthcare professionals and their families, friends or carers.

Adults with type 1 diabetes are offered a structured education programme 6–12 months after diagnosis. One such structured education programme is DAFNE (Dose Adjustment For Normal Eating), which aims to help adults with type 1 diabetes lead as normal a life as possible, whilst also maintaining blood glucose levels within healthy targets in order to reduce the risk of long-term diabetes complications (Figure 8.1).

Core education topics

Insulin therapy

Most people with type 1 diabetes are offered multiple daily injections or basal-bolus insulin regimens as opposed to mixed insulin. A basal-bolus regimen consists of rapid-acting insulin (bolus) at mealtimes and long-acting (basal) insulin once or twice a day, which roughly replicates how a person's pancreas normally delivers insulin. Although a basal-bolus regimen involves more insulin injections each day, it allows for flexibility as to when meals are taken and omission of rapid-acting insulin if eating a carbohydrate-free meal. Individuals are taught how to inject

Diabetes Care at a Glance, First Edition. Edited by Anne Phillips.
© 2023 John Wiley & Sons Ltd. Published 2023 by John Wiley & Sons Ltd.

insulin using insulin pens, with some switching to an insulin pump after a while. Those who find a basal-bolus regimen difficult to use may find a mixed insulin pen easier.

Dietary advice

People are advised to avoid buying foods labelled 'diabetic' and make healthy food choices that are lower in saturated fat, sugar and salt. Doing this will help to control blood fats and blood pressure, maintain a healthy weight and reduce diabetes complications. A good diet provides maximum nutrition while allowing the intake of carbohydrates, protein and fat to be monitored. Talking to a dietitian is an important part of type 1 diabetes education. Dietitians help improve understanding of how diet affects diabetes and consider the options available, and then plan changes individuals can make to achieve their goals. This expert advice is designed to suit different lifestyles, any other health problems and any cultural preferences.

Carbohydrate counting

Carbohydrates are the main part of the diet that affect blood glucose levels and carbohydrate counting is a key skill in managing blood glucose levels. This helps people to match their rapid-acting insulin to their meals and snacks and reduces the chances of severe increases and decreases in their glucose levels. If someone matches their mealtime insulin to their meals, their blood glucose levels will be in target by the next meal. Some individuals on fixed doses of mealtime insulin but who eat variable amounts of carbohydrates at mealtimes could find it difficult, without carbohydrate counting, to manage their blood glucose levels as different carbohydrate foods vary in their impact on blood glucose levels.

The basic principle of carbohydrate counting is that 10 g of carbohydrates raise blood glucose levels by 2–3 mmol/l and 1 unit of rapid-acting insulin lowers blood glucose by 2–3 mmol/l. Based on this, individuals beginning carbohydrate counting will often start with an insulin to carbohydrate ratio of 1 g of insulin for every 10 g of carbohydrates. There are several resources that people can access to improve their skills and confidence in estimating foods by eye if they do not have access to food labels.

Blood glucose monitoring

Everyone with type 1 diabetes needs to monitor their blood glucose levels and HbA1c to keep their diabetes on track, which reduces the risk of developing complications. Testing provides a better understanding of how different foods and activities impact on blood glucose levels. Blood glucose levels can be measured by a fingerprick test or by using continuous glucose monitoring (CGM) or flash glucose monitoring. More details on CGM and flash monitoring can be found in Chapter 19. Every person will have their set targets for blood glucose which they agree with their diabetes team. Hypoglycaemia management is also discussed.

Physical activity

Education also includes information on the benefits of physical activity for blood glucose, blood pressure and weight control and so relevant information should be given on appropriate activity for the individual. An important issue is the individual's understanding of the impact of activity on blood glucose control and their ability to develop knowledge and skills to avoid hypoglycaemia and hyperglycaemia. Therefore, they need to learn how to adjust their insulin doses and carbohydrate intake prior to, during and after exercise. Guidelines suggest that people with diabetes perform 150 minutes of physical activity per week, which could consist of 30 minutes of moderate activity five days a week. Exercising at moderate intensity, one should be able to talk to others without gasping for air.

References

Kiddell, C., Ryan, L., and Kelly, C. (2019). A STEP forward: delivering structured education from the day of diagnosis of type 1 diabetes. *J. Diabet. Nurs.* 23: JDN068.

National Institute for Health and Care Excellence (2022). Type 1 Diabetes in Adults: Diagnosis and Management. NICE Guideline NG17. Available at www.nice.org.uk/guidance/ng17.

9 Structured education in type 2 diabetes

Figure 9.1 Preventable long-term complications of diabetes.

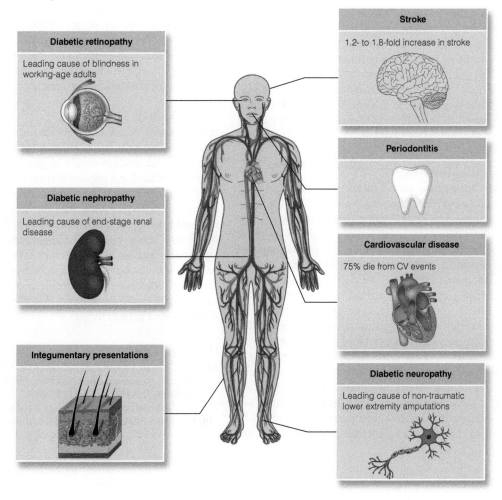

Diabetic retinopathy

Leading cause of blindness in working-age adults

Diabetic nephropathy

Leading cause of end-stage renal disease

Integumentary presentations

Stroke

1.2- to 1.8-fold increase in stroke

Periodontitis

Cardiovascular disease

75% die from CV events

Diabetic neuropathy

Leading cause of non-traumatic lower extremity amputations

Figure 9.2 Fundamentals of structured education.

- Education based on principles of adult learning
- Education from a trained multidisciplinary team
- Education should be assessable to a broad range of people inclusive of cultural awareness, ethnicity, disability and geographical location.
- Education should use a variety of techniques to promote active learning, and should be adapted to meet individuals needs, choices and learning styles.
- Education should be integrated into routine diabetes care.
- Education should be available to everyone with diabetes.

Figure 9.3 The aims of all structured education.

- Explore signs and symptoms
- The potential for dietary change
- The benefits of engagement in physical activity
- The benefits of weight loss
- Role of medications

Diabetes Care at a Glance, First Edition. Edited by Anne Phillips.
© 2023 John Wiley & Sons Ltd. Published 2023 by John Wiley & Sons Ltd.

The diagnosis of diabetes can be devastating and many individuals can be left in a state of shock, especially if the diagnosis was unexpected. In addition, they can go on to feel overwhelmed by the burden of information and appointments. Providing a structured education programme for people with type 2 diabetes is very important as this will enable a greater understanding of what diabetes is but will also provide a greater awareness of the practical lifestyle steps they can take to support self-management, improve glycaemic control and improve their quality of life. The achievement of good glycaemic control helps to minimize the long-term microvascular and macrovascular complications (Figure 9.1), the development of which will not only have a detrimental effect on a person's quality of life but will also impose increased costs on the NHS for their treatment.

The access to structured education for people with diabetes is fully covered in the National Institute for Health and Care Excellence (NICE 2022) clinical guidelines for the management of type 2 diabetes (NG28). Structured education is recommended from the point of diagnosis with annual review (see Chapter 29) and encourages people with type 2 diabetes to recognize that diabetes education needs to be at the centre of their approach to self-management of their diabetes.

Health literacy and numeracy refers to the capacity to obtain, process and understand basic health information with which to make a decision relating to lifestyle choices. This has significant implications for health educators and the delivery of structured education for diabetes. Research has shown that there is a relationship between individuals with suboptimal levels of literacy and limited knowledge pertaining to their diabetes. In addition, research has shown an association between diabetes-related numeracy skills and an individual's glycaemic control. This does not mean that people with modest health literacy cannot learn, but the learning needs to be delivered in innovative ways to inform them about their diabetes and expectations.

There has been much positive evidence of the benefits of structured education. Education is an effective catalyst for biomedical and psychological benefits, but the length of follow-up and variable generalizability of the findings of various programmes available makes it difficult to assess their wide-ranging application. Effective education goes beyond the passive relay of information to a more intensive coaching that results in behaviour change and an opportunity for improved health status over time. This makes it clear that there must be a long-term investment to ensure that participants not only understand the information given but can also apply it, and that it has long-term benefits.

In structured education for people with type 2 diabetes, four critical areas to support self-management have been introduced into structured education programmes to support attitudes, beliefs, knowledge and skills for the learner, their family and carers (Figure 9.2). There are two nationally recognized programmes of structured education for type 2 diabetes:
- Diabetes Education and Self-Management for Ongoing and Newly Diagnosed (DESMOND)
- X-PERT.

Additionally, many hospital trusts and clinical commissioning groups have developed their own locally delivered structured education programmes rather than adopting DESMOND or X-PERT. The aim of all structured education programmes for people with type 2 diabetes is to encourage self-empowerment and self-management in order to provide the optimum quality of life achievable by the individual alone (Figure 9.3).

Research on the effectiveness of diabetes education using DESMOND, compared with standard care, has shown greater improvements in weight loss and smoking cessation, and positive improvements in illness beliefs, but no difference in HbA1c levels up to 12 months after diagnosis. Interestingly, at the three-year follow-up no difference was noted for biomedical and lifestyle outcomes or medication use, but significant benefits relating to illness beliefs were sustained.

The National Diabetes Audit (2018) showed that whilst 91% of people with type 2 diabetes are offered structured education, only 8.2% were recorded as having attended. It is important not to assume that people will automatically attend diabetes education following a referral from the GP practice just because it is beneficial for them. A discussion about the education referral is needed if there is to be a joint agreement to the referral being made. In addition, all healthcare providers involved in diabetes care and education providers need to promote the content and benefits of the education and identify any additional support that people may need to ensure their attendance.

Whilst it is apparent that structured diabetes education can create a beneficial effect in terms of health benefits, further research is opportune to test the effects on prolonged glycaemic control. No one individual education programme can and will meet the needs of people with diabetes, but the programme can establish the first layer of understanding for partnership working and individualized care approaches to augment and scaffold thereafter. The challenges of Covid-19 has changed the way in which education programmes are being delivered and is providing more choice in the future to include face-to-face group education and virtual group education online.

References
National Diabetes Audit (2018). National Diabetes Audit 2016–17. Report 1: Care Processes and Treatment Targets. www.hqip.org.uk/wp-content/uploads/2018/03/National-Diabetes-Audit-2016-17-Report-1-Care-Processes-and-Treatment-T.pdf.
National Institute for Health and Care Excellence (2022). Type 2 Diabetes in Adults: Management. NICE Guideline NG28. www.nice.org.uk/guidance/ng28.

10 Information prescriptions

Figure 10.1 Diabetes UK information prescriptions for healthcare professionals. *Source:* The British Diabetic Association operating as Diabetes UK; https://www.diabetes.org.uk/professionals/resources/resources-to-improve-your-clinical-practice/information-prescriptions-qa.

Blood pressure	PDF, 36 KB	Word, 1.5 MB
Cholesterol	PDF, 35 KB	Word, 1.4 MB
HbA1c	PDF, 40 KB	Word, 1.5 MB
Type 2 diabetes remission	PDF, 50 KB	Word, 2.3MB
Emotions	PDF, 33 KB	Word, 1.1 MB
Improving your diabetes knowledge	PDF, 45 KB	Word, 2 MB
Keeping your kidneys healthy	PDF, 34 KB	Word, 1.5 MB
Kidney disease	PDF, 33 KB	Word, 1.5 MB
Contraception and pregnancy	PDF, 34 KB	Word, 1.5 MB
Feet (low risk)	PDF, 53 KB	Word, 1.4 MB
Feet (moderate/high risk)	PDF, 54 KB	Word, 1.4 MB

Figure 10.2 Diabetes UK information prescription about improving diabetes knowledge for people with diabetes. *Source:* The British Diabetic Association operating as Diabetes UK.

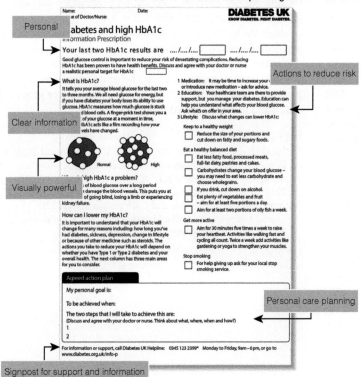

Figure 10.3 Diabetes and high HbA1c information prescription. *Source:* The British Diabetic Association operating as Diabetes UK.

Diabetes Care at a Glance, First Edition. Edited by Anne Phillips.
© 2023 John Wiley & Sons Ltd. Published 2023 by John Wiley & Sons Ltd.

Diabetes UK have produced and designed useful online resources known as information prescriptions. These are a downloadable resource with easy-to-read accessible information on one A4 page (Figure 10.1). The information prescriptions are available in themes (Figure 10.2) and are designed to be used in consultation conversations to make every contact count and share useful information. Information prescriptions are designed to be used by health professionals when consulting with people with diabetes to help them understand and improve their health targets and manage their diabetes.

Information prescriptions allow people to receive accessible information and record their latest test results, with an explanation of what these mean for the individual concerned. They can also offer an opportunity to set person-centred and individualized goals and identify steps for people with diabetes to take to help improve their diabetes and health.

Information prescriptions matter because they offer individualized support in a personal document that is easy to read and is short. They have a national reach and are embedded in all primary care diabetes systems and services. They help in the fight against complications and offer clinically accurate information to help people with diabetes gain awareness of how to prevent complications. They also offer an opportunity to transform care and support care planning and behaviour change to support self-care.

General practitioners and practice nurses report that information prescriptions put people with diabetes 'in the driving seat' and that this is key in supporting successful behaviour change and are thus a really useful patient resource. After the introduction of information prescriptions into routine diabetes and pre-diabetes care in one Scottish GP practice, audit found a 10% reduction in patients reaching their HbA1c targets. In Manchester, after the introduction of kidney health information prescriptions, regular practice audit reported improved management of patients with diabetes and renal disease and less prescription of contraindicated antidiabetic medications.

Figure 10.2 details the types of resource that are available to download for people with diabetes. The three core information prescriptions that influence someone's risk of complications include those on blood pressure, cholesterol and HbA1c. Unfortunately, only 36% of people with diabetes achieve the targets recommended by the National Institute for Health and Care Excellence (2022a,b). People with levels outside of these targets are at higher risk of blindness, renal failure, amputation, myocardial infarction and stroke.

Information prescriptions are needed as the UK spends over £8 billion annually treating preventable complications (Baxter et al. 2016) and this cost is predicted to increase to nearly £17 billion if interventions are not established. Information prescriptions can be a quick and effective tool for engaging people in their diabetes care, allowing individuals to increase control of their health and understanding of their condition. Diabetes UK report that more than 100 000 information prescriptions have been saved on individual health records, with over 35 000 individual access requests by people with diabetes.

As can be seen in Figure 10.3 the information prescription is designed to be easy to use. First, personal information is entered to create ownership, followed by documentation of results for HbA1c, cholesterol, blood pressure or weight. Clear information follows, using easy everyday language and avoiding medical jargon. The images are visually powerful to also engage visual learners. The individualized actions to reduce risk follow, and the last section comprises the agreed action plan and goals, which are signed and dated. Signposts at the bottom of the information prescription indicate further information and support.

References

Baxter, M., Hudson, R., Mahon, J. et al. (2016). Estimating the impact of better management of glycaemic control in adults with type 1 and type 2 diabetes on the number of clinical complications and the associated financial benefit. *Diabet. Med.* 33 (11): 1575–1581. https://doi.org/10.1111/dme.13062.

National Institute of Health and Care Excellence (2022a). Type 1 Diabetes in Adults: Diagnosis and Management. NICE Guideline NG17. https://www.nice.org.uk/guidance/ng17.

National Institute of Health and Care Excellence (2022b). Type 2 Diabetes in Adults: Management. NICE Guideline NG28. www.nice.org.uk/guidance/ng28.

11 Emotional and psychological support

Figure 11.1 The grief cycle of Elizabeth Kübler-Ross (1969).

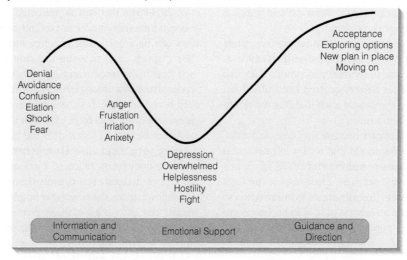

Denial
Avoidance
Confusion
Elation
Shock
Fear

Anger
Frustation
Irriation
Anixety

Depression
Overwhelmed
Helplessness
Hostility
Fight

Acceptance
Exploring options
New plan in place
Moving on

Information and Communication

Emotional Support

Guidance and Direction

Figure 11.2 Diabetes UK 7As model.

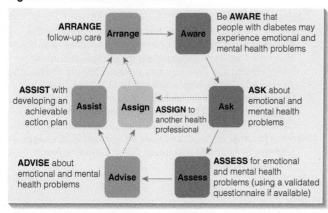

ARRANGE follow-up care — Arrange

Aware — Be **AWARE** that people with diabetes may experience emotional and mental health problems

ASSIST with developing an achievable action plan — Assist

Assign — **ASSIGN** to another health professional

Ask — **ASK** about emotional and mental health problems

ADVISE about emotional and mental health problems — Advise

Assess — **ASSESS** for emotional and mental health problems (using a validated questionnaire if available)

Figure 11.3 iDEAL diabetes consultation checklist.

LET'S TALK NOW!

iDEAL
Insights for Diabetes Excellence, Access and Learning
www.idealdiabetes.com
@iDEALdiabetes

What do I want to know today about my diabetes?

What do I want to talk about in my diabetes appointment today?

What are my latest test results and what do they mean?

How am I feeling about having diabetes?

Do I have any questions I would like answered?

Diabetes is known as one of the most psychologically and behaviourally demanding conditions to live with. Diabetes can be relentless and requires constant attention, awareness and decision-making. Hendrieckx et al. (2019) found that 64% of people sometimes or often felt depressed because of their diabetes. Also, less than 25% of people are able to access the emotional and psychological help they need from the NHS. Glucose fluctuations, from hypoglycaemia (low glucose) to hyperglycaemia (high glucose), also have major effects on mood and brain function (Holt et al. 2014).

People with diabetes often report feelings of fear, anger, resentment and devastation at their diagnosis and often experience feelings like the grief cycle, originally described in a landmark work by Kübler-Ross (1969). People with diabetes can experience the stages of grief at diagnosis or during the lifespan of diabetes when treatment escalation is required or a complication is diagnosed. The five stages are denial, anger, bargaining, depression and acceptance (Figure 11.1).

People may be anxious about their annual review and consider it a stressful rather than helpful experience as this is when a deterioration in their diabetes management is discovered or a new complication is diagnosed. Practitioners need to be mindful of this and not assume our approaches are seen as helpful by the individuals we work alongside.

As discussed in Chapter 4 about the power and impact of language and the words we use in diabetes care, the communication we share with people living with diabetes can and does have a profound effect. Enforced changes to an individual's lifestyle necessitated by diabetes can impact on an individual's well-being and cause feelings of 'loss of control'. This can be psychologically and emotionally disabling, causing 'diabetes distress'. Helpful guides for people with diabetes are available to support their adjustment to diabetes, and local support groups can be useful additions. Diabetes UK and the Australian Centre for Behavioural Research in Diabetes have created excellent resources to help practitioners working with people with diabetes to discuss their emotional needs and to use consultation conversations more effectively (Hendrieckx et al. 2019). Diabetes UK's 7As model (Figure 11.2) offers a series of stages to follow, backed up by the resources in the practical guide, that are invaluable in supporting emotional and physical health and providing holistic care. The 7As model for assessment of diabetes distress comprises the following stages: Aware, Ask, Assess, Advise, Assist, Assign and Arrange. This system is designed to be flexible and to help direct people to the most appropriate services as required. To identify diabetes distress, health professionals should be aware, ask and assess each individual to enable them to be heard and feel understood.

People with diabetes are twice as likely to experience depression and are more likely to experience it for longer. The psychological stressors involved in living with diabetes can include fear of injections and treatments, fear or experience of hypoglycaemia, eating disorders, focus on weight and having to be weighed at each diabetes review, and the distress caused by the perceived misunderstandings of others. People with diabetes can also feel judged by practitioners and this can create mistrust and emotional distress.

People with diabetes can prepare for their consultation conversations by recording what they want to ask so that they feel they have a voice in their diabetes care. The use of a preparation checklist can be helpful in guiding the conversation to the needs of the person (Figure 11.3). These are useful as part of holistic diabetes care and give ownership to people with diabetes for their consultation conversations.

Living with diabetes is a dynamic process that can change due to triggers such as a new impairment or treatment changes. These changes can trigger sorrow or a loss of control if the person has experienced an unexpected hypo for example. Loss of independence and spontaneity can cause distress as diabetes does require rigorous planning and attention to detail, which can cause frustration – this requires understanding and patience.

References

Hendrieckx, C., Halliday, J.A., Beeney, L., and Speight, J. (2019). *Diabetes and emotional health: a practical guide for healthcare professionals supporting adults with type 1 and type 2 diabetes*, 2e. London: Diabetes UK.
Holt, R.I.G., de Groot, M., and Golden, S.H. (2014). Diabetes and depression. *Curr. Diab. Rep.* 14 (6): 491. https://doi.org/10.1007/s11892-014-0491-3.
Kübler-Ross, E. (1969). *On Death and Dying*. New York: Macmillan.

12 Person-centred goal setting and assessing risk

Figure 12.1 Goal setting: three essential components.

1. Goal identification
2. Setting the goal(s)
3. Monitoring, feedback and encouragement

Figure 12.2 A decision balance sheet.

	Disadvantages	Advantages
No Change		
Change		

Figure 12.3 Scaling tool.

On a scale of 1–10, how important is it for you to make this change?
(0 = unimportant, 10 = very important)

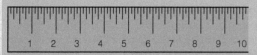

1 2 3 4 5 6 7 8 9 10

Importance =

Tip: if it's 7 or above, it suggests it is important enough to you for it to be really worth making this change

Figure 12.4 SMARTER acronym.

S	Specific	Clearly define the goal: 'I am going to take more exercise' is not specific. 'I'm going to take a walk every day during my lunch-hour starting with 15 minutes and increasing by 5 minutes every three days until I reach 30 minutes' walk every day' is a specific goal
M	Measurable	This shows the progress towards the goal for example and whether it has been achieved
A	Achievable	This should be explored from the individual's point of view and check the timeframe for the goal also to ensure it is possible and realistic for the person who has chosen it
R	Realistic	Goals must be realistic. While a 2 stone weight loss is achievable and possible, to say this will happen in a month is not realistic
T	Timed	Goals are more likely to be undertaken if a specific time is set for them in terms of the day and as in S in terms of the time of day also (lunchtime)
E	Evaluate	Evaluate goals regularly and adjust as needed to consider any changes needed. This also gives ownership to the persons whose goal (s) it is or they are and offers encouragement to increase their goals when they have achieved the original goal (s) set
R	Recorded	Record the goal setting decision using an Information Prescription and also keep a copy in the health professional records so it can be referred back on in subsequent clinical conversation as required

f it was easy to change behaviours there would be far fewer people around the world living with or at risk of long-term conditions such as diabetes or cardiovascular diseases. The International Diabetes Federation (IDF 2021) reported that 'Diabetes must be taken seriously not only by individuals living with, or at high risk of the condition but also by healthcare professionals and policy makers.' It is vital for people with diabetes to be supported through person-centred and individualized education to learn to live with diabetes successfully to improve their health and well-being. Person-centred approaches to diabetes care and placing the individual at the heart of their health and care planning supports self-management as a core component. People with diabetes can feel more supported and confident if they are encouraged in this by health professionals (Furze and Phillips 2017).

When a condition like diabetes develops, people can equate the severity of the condition with 'symptom load' – if someone has symptoms, then they can consider their condition as 'severe'. However, as people learn to live with their diabetes, the perceived severity can lessen and their quality of life can improve. However, health professionals cannot assume that those with the worst symptoms or worst perceived quality of life will have the most severe illness, nor can it be assumed that people with the perceived most severe forms of diabetes with perhaps advanced complications will have a poorer quality of life. These observations are at the core of person-centred care – supporting self-management must start where the person reports that he or she is, not where we as health professionals think the person should be according to HbA1c results for example.

Goal setting and pacing can be a good way to avoid the overactivity–rest trap while supporting continuing health change. Furze et al. (2008) suggested helping people to slowly increase their activities, for example physical activity, with the aim of maintenance and gradual improvement in order to avoid early over-exertion and failure. The evidence for self-management interventions that include goal setting as a core skill shows that people have reduced symptoms, increased understanding, reduced anxiety and depression, and increased perceptions of control, fitness and quality of life (Furze and Phillips 2017).

Goal setting with individuals comprises three essential steps (Figure 12.1). The choice of goal to target for behaviour change must always lie with the individual it concerns. At the same time the person needs to also decide at which point the goal will be reached by setting a realistic and achievable time frame. Information prescriptions can assist in the individual goal-setting process (see Chapter 10). This can be frustrating for health professionals as we may perceive a goal to be more health promoting (i.e. stopping smoking), but for the goal to be successful it has to be owned by the individual it concerns. When introducing goal setting, listing the pros and cons using a decision balance sheet simply drawn on a piece of paper can be a useful approach (Figure 12.2) so individuals can see the potential benefits. When someone with diabetes has one or two health decisions to make, calling them goals can focus the person's attention to their goal.

Using scaling questions on how important the goal is to the individual can also be helpful. For example, by asking how confident the person is in achieving their goal, with 1 being not confident and 10 being very confident, you will see how much self-belief the individual has in their goal (Figure 12.3). If the goal is less important to the person, you can try to increase their motivation towards that goal; however, if the individual perceives the goal as unimportant, behaviour change is likely to be unsuccessful. Once a confidence score reaches 7, the goal is more likely to be successful.

The SMARTER acronym (Figure 12.4) can guide the person to the detail and time scale involved in achieving their goal. Supporting each individual with diabetes to anticipate potential difficulties and how to deal with these increases the chances of their success (Furze and Phillips 2017). Providing positive feedback to people with diabetes can offer encouragement when they need to make behaviour changes and set goals. For healthcare professionals to understand the importance of this will help people with diabetes to feel supported and enabled.

References

Furze, G. and Phillips, A. (2017). Goal setting: a key skill for person-centred care. In: *Principles of Diabetes Care: An Essential Guide for Health Professionals* (ed. A. Phillips), chapter 7. Salisbury: Quay Books.

Furze, G., Donnison, J., and Lewin, R. (2008). *The Clinician's Guide to Chronic Disease Management for Long Term Conditions: A Cognitive Behavioural Approach*. Keswick: M&K Update Ltd.

International Diabetes Federation (2021). *IDF Diabetes Atlas*, 10e. https://diabetesatlas.org/idfawp/resource-files/2021/07/IDF_Atlas_10th_Edition_2021.pdf.

Partnership working and adjustment to living with diabetes

Figure 13.1 Partnerships in healthcare.

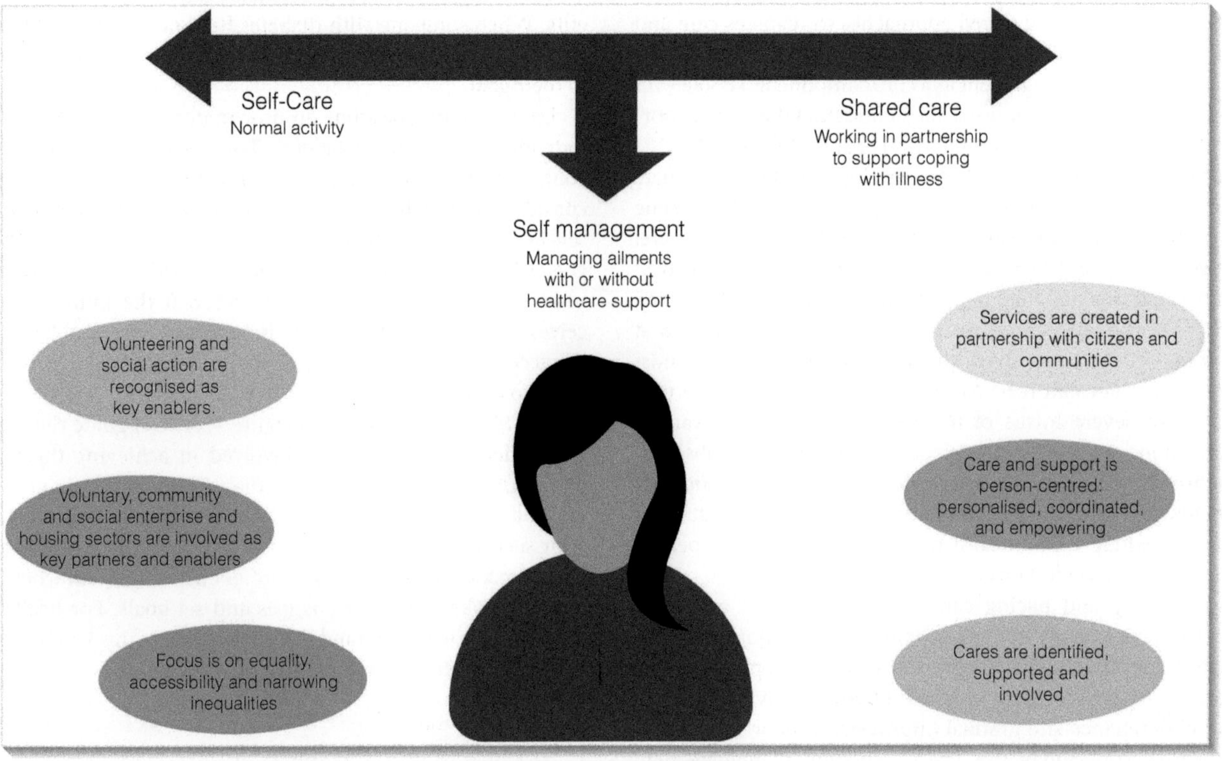

Self-Care
Normal activity

Shared care
Working in partnership
to support coping
with illness

Self management
Managing ailments
with or without
healthcare support

Volunteering and
social action are
recognised as
key enablers.

Voluntary, community
and social enterprise and
housing sectors are involved as
key partners and enablers

Focus is on equality,
accessibility and narrowing
inequalities

Services are created in
partnership with citizens and
communities

Care and support is
person-centred:
personalised, coordinated,
and empowering

Cares are identified,
supported and
involved

Figure 13.2 Person with diabetes at the centre of their care. *Source:* Williams and Pickup (1999).

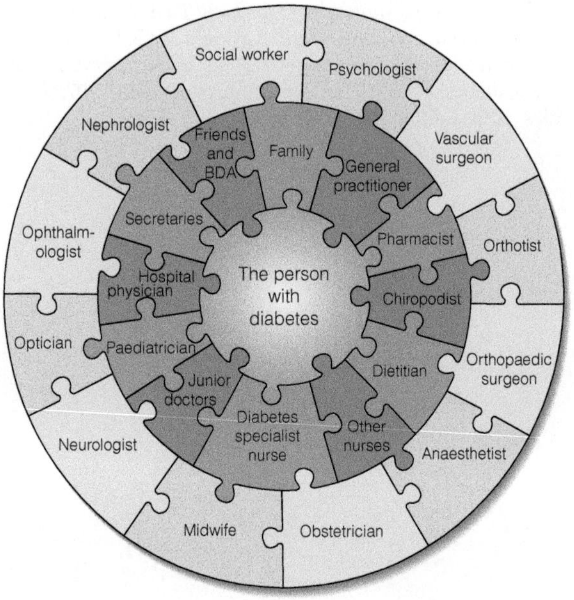

Social worker
Psychologist
Nephrologist
Friends and BDA
Family
General practitioner
Vascular surgeon
Secretaries
Pharmacist
Orthotist
Ophthalmologist
Hospital physician
The person with diabetes
Chiropodist
Optician
Paediatrician
Dietitian
Orthopaedic surgeon
Junior doctors
Neurologist
Diabetes specialist nurse
Other nurses
Anaesthetist
Midwife
Obstetrician

Figure 13.3 Partnership working.

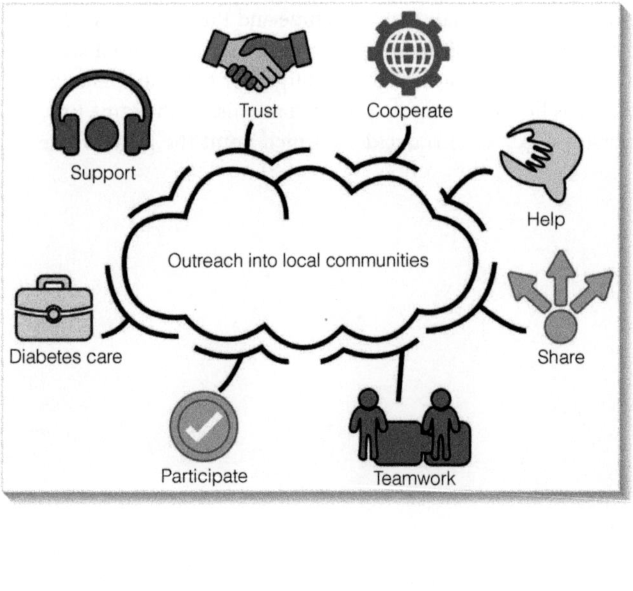

Trust
Cooperate
Support
Help
Outreach into local communities
Diabetes care
Share
Participate
Teamwork

Diabetes Care at a Glance, First Edition. Edited by Anne Phillips.
© 2023 John Wiley & Sons Ltd. Published 2023 by John Wiley & Sons Ltd.

Living with diabetes can be psychologically and emotionally challenging for individuals newly diagnosed, and indeed for people diagnosed for many years (see Chapter 11). Building effective partnerships between healthcare professionals and individuals and their families can provide the supportive care to which many people positively respond.

Good patient–provider communication (see Chapter 4) and shared decision-making (see Chapter 12) has been positively associated with improved diabetes self-management and glycaemic control in people with diabetes (Rouyard et al. 2021). Using a person-centred and individualized approach with every individual with diabetes can be beneficial in producing a plan to promote self-care and learning, starting from the point of diagnosis or from a change in a health condition so that adaptation and acceptance of the new health status can be supported.

The Health Foundation (2022) has for many years developed person-centred and partnership tools to help practitioners to develop partnership approaches. As shown in Figure 13.1, outreach into local communities and social partnership approaches can also respond to people's requirements.

Health is multifaceted and many different dimensions of wellness and health contribute to each person's holistic health. Being diagnosed with diabetes or a complication of diabetes can damage the sense of wellness and requires every person to draw on their inner resolve to adapt to this change in their lives. Accordingly, having practitioners who are enablers and who work in partnerships can support people to make this acclimatization to their lives. This is an essential role in diabetes care: to 'walk alongside the individual' offering support, being non-judgemental and affirming of people's life choices in a guided way (see Chapters 10–12).

A range of different healthcare professionals cooperate to provide care for people with diabetes who should be at the centre of their care (Figure 13.2). These healthcare professionals may work at a diabetes specialist centre within a hospital outpatient department or on a ward that cares for people with diabetes or within primary care.

Respecting cultural and spiritual beliefs and reaching out to learn about local populations can also enable partnerships to grow and trust to be facilitated. The prevalence of diabetes in minority ethnic communitiesis alarmingly high, approximately three to five times higher than the white British population (Goff 2019). Particularly striking is the earlier onset of type 2 diabetes (some 10–12 years younger), with a significant proportion of individuals being diagnosed before the age of 40. Goff (2019) suggested that this could be due to a complex interplay of biological, lifestyle, social, clinical and healthcare system factors that are known to drive these health disparities. Furthermore, evidence suggests that the hardest-to-reach vulnerable populations with high diabetes incidence or risk also experience health disparities that lead to fewer medication reviews and slower escalation of diabetes prescribing as required (Phillips 2021). Evidence also underpins the debates about reconsidering diabetes services, promoting effective partnership working and in particular listening and working with local practices and their communities to share diabetes health messages and provide accessible and appropriate diabetes person-centred education opportunities (Phillips 2021).

Teamworking and partnership enabling is synergistically effective (Figure 13.3) and many positive health- and diabetes-related outcomes can be achieved through partnership working across traditional health boundaries. Encouraging team building, sharing contacts and reaching out to build partnerships can help people with diabetes to gain health and social support. People with diabetes should be encouraged to access the relevant voluntary agencies and charity groups that can also offer social support.

Intuitive diabetes care and practitioners who have intuition or who can develop their intuitive approaches can go beyond the spoken words and create partnerships with people with diabetes, in particular reaching out to the most vulnerable and hardest to reach to enable access and equity in diabetes education and services. Establishing trust and forming partnerships across diabetes care with local communities can be the pivotal catalyst to help people gain their sense of well-being, control and self-management skills through their life journey with diabetes.

References

Goff, L. (2019). Ethnicity and type 2 diabetes in the UK. *Diabet. Med.* 36 (8): 927–938. https://doi.org/10.1111/dme.13895.

Phillips, A. (2021). Diabetes care: a time to review prescribing approaches and reach out into local communities. *J. Prescr. Pract.* 3 (5): 2–8.

Rouyard, T., Leal, J., Salvi, D., et al. (2021). An intuitive risk communication tool to enhance patient–provider partnership in diabetes consultation. *J. Diabetes Sci.Technol.* 16(4): 988–994. https://doi.org/10.1177/1932296821995800.

The Health Foundation (2022). Our Partnerships. www.health.org.uk/funding-and-partnerships/our-partnerships

Williams, G. and Pickup, J. (1999). *Handbook of Diabetes Care*, 2e, 208. Oxford: Wiley Blackwell.

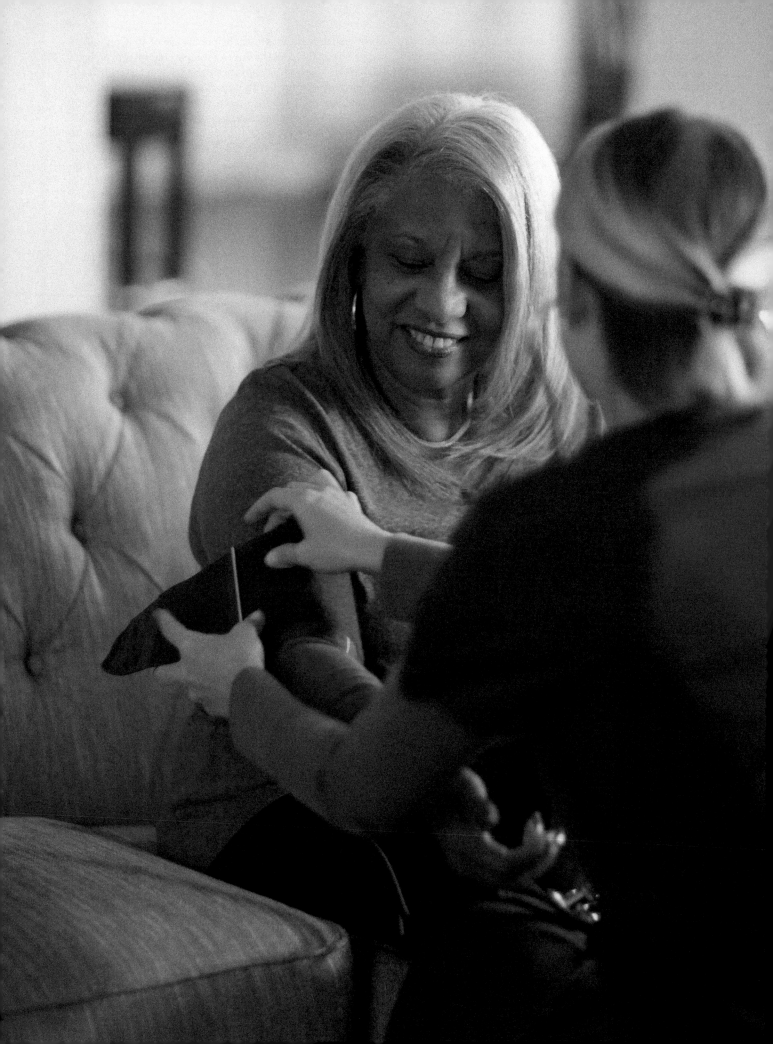

Pharmacological treatments

Part 3

Chapters

14 Oral antidiabetic medications

Figure 14.1 Summary of characteristics of drugs used in type 2 diabetes. *Source:* Stewart (2021), Adapted from Tahrani et al. (2016) and GPNotebook Education (2020).

Class	Examples	Physiological action	Cautions	Hypoglycaemia risk	Weight change	Cost
Biguanides	Metformin hydrochloride	» Decreases hepatic glucose production » Increases insulin sensitivity	» Gastrointestinal side effects » Contraindicated at estimated glomerular filtration rate (eGFR) <30 mL/min	No	Neutral	Low
Sulphonylureas	Gliclazide Glipizide	» Increases insulin secretion	» Risk of hypoglycaemia	Yes	Gain	Low
Thiazolidinediones	Pioglitazone	» Increases insulin sensitivity	» Bladder cancer » Bone fractures » Oedema » Heart failure	No	Gain	Low
Glucagon-like peptide-1 (GLP-1) analogues	Semaglutide	» Slows gastric emptying » Reduces appetite » Stimulates insulin release	» Pancreatitis	No	Loss	High
Dipeptidyl peptidase-4 (DPP-4) inhibitors	Sitagliptin Saxagliptin Alogliptin Linagliptin	» Blocks DPP-4, which is an enzyme that inactivates GLP-1 » Increase GLP-1 levels	» Pancreatitis	No	Neutral	High
Sodium-glucose cotransporter-2 (SGLT2) inhibitors	Empagliflozin Canagliflozin Dapagliflozin	» Inhibits renal glucose reabsorption	» Urinary tract infection » Candidiasis (thrush) » Euglycaemic diabetic ketoacidosis » Avoid in active foot disease	No	Loss	High

The different medications developed for type 2 diabetes are aimed at tackling issues including obesity, reduced insulin production, insulin resistance, dysfunction of digestive hormones, increased glucose production by the liver and cardiovascular complications (Tahrani et al. 2016; National Institute for Health and Care Excellence 2022). The different classes of drugs, how they work (mode of action), and the associated cautions and side effects are presented in Figure 14.1.

Sulfonylureas

Sulfonylureas (SUs) include gliclazide and glipizide.

Mode of action
SUs stimulate the beta cells in the pancreas to release insulin.

Advantages
Low cost and rapid onset of action to lower blood glucose levels in the treatment of symptomatic hyperglycaemia. SUs are also the first-choice tablet for steroid-induced hyperglycaemia (see Chapter 25).

Cautions and side effects
Since SUs stimulate insulin secretion, even in the presence of low blood glucose levels, they can cause hypoglycaemia (very low blood glucose levels). Therefore, people starting an SU require education about blood glucose monitoring and hypoglycaemia management. People whose kidneys are functioning poorly and those at risk of falls may not be suitable for an SU because they are at risk of hypoglycaemia. People can also gain up to 4 kg in weight, so it may put people off these drugs.

Metformin

Mode of action
Metformin slows down excess glucose release by the liver, reducing glucose in the blood. It also diminishes insulin resistance, making the muscle and fat cells sensitive to insulin.

Advantages
It does not cause hypoglycaemia when used on its own, and is weight-neutral (does not cause weight gain or loss).

Cautions and side effects
Metformin should be avoided in people with poor kidney function, i.e. when estimated glomerular filtration rate (eGFR) is below 30 ml/min. Metformin should be stopped during illness if there is an increased risk of dehydration, but should be restarted when patients have recovered. Common side effects include nausea, vomiting and diarrhoea, and these will be lessened if metformin is taken with a meal; alternatively, patients may need slow-release metformin.

Diabetes Care at a Glance, First Edition. Edited by Anne Phillips.
© 2023 John Wiley & Sons Ltd. Published 2023 by John Wiley & Sons Ltd.

Sodium/glucose cotransporter-2 inhibitors

Examples include empagliflozin, canagliflozin and dapagliflozin.

Mode of action

These drugs encourage the kidneys to excrete excess glucose through urine. Normally, the kidneys filter up to 180 g/day of glucose and most of it is reabsorbed into the body and reused. This reabsorption is controlled by proteins in the kidneys called sodium/glucose cotransporter-2 (SGLT2). SGLT2 inhibitors prevent excess glucose from being reabsorbed, resulting in blood glucose levels decreasing to normal levels.

Advantages

There is a low risk of hypoglycaemia because these drugs do not affect the pancreas and can promote weight loss of around 2–3 kg over three months by the loss of calories in urine. Recent studies have shown that SGLT2 inhibitors can benefit people with cardiac and renal conditions, which can be long-term complications of diabetes.

Cautions and side effects

There is a risk of dehydration and kidney injury if taken during serious illness. When people with type 2 diabetes are admitted to hospital, it is advised that they stop their SGLT2 inhibitors until they are well and discharged. Passing sugary urine can cause urine infections and thrush so some people have to stop taking them.

Thiazolidinediones

Pioglitazone is the only thiazolidinedione (TZD).

Mode of action

Like metformin, it is an insulin sensitizer, so it helps muscle and fat cells to become more sensitive to insulin and reduces the amount of glucose released by the liver. It may take one week for a notable reduction in blood glucose levels and 4–12 weeks to take full effect.

Advantages

Low cost and low hypoglycaemia risk.

Cautions and side effects

TZDs should be avoided in patients with bladder cancer, where there is a higher risk of fractures, or in congestive heart failure. There is also weight gain of 2–3 kg.

Glucagon-like peptide 1 analogues

Injectable examples include liraglutide (Victoza), semaglutide (Ozempic) and dulaglutide (Trulicity). The only current oral GLP-1 is semaglutide (Rybelsus).

Mode of action

Glucagon-like peptide 1 (GLP-1) is a natural hormone released by the intestines in response to eating, and people with type 2 diabetes do not produce enough. The GPL-1 that humans produce is inactivated after two minutes by an enzyme called dipeptidyl peptidase 4 (DPP-4). GLP-1 analogues mimic the action of natural GLP-1, increasing the duration of action of natural GLP-1. They increase insulin release by the pancreas only when food is eaten, so there is a low risk of hypoglycaemia. They also reduce the amount of glucose released by the liver. GLP-1 analogues slow the movement of food through the gut and the individual feels full sooner than usual. This means an individual eats less and can lose up to 6 kg in weight with certain of these drugs.

Cautions and side effects

Vomiting and diarrhoea, although these tend to reduce over time.

Dipeptidyl peptidase 4 inhibitors

Examples include sitagliptin, saxagliptin, alogliptin and linagliptin.

Mode of action

DPP-4 inhibitors block DPP-4 from inactivating GLP-1 in type 2 diabetes. As a result, the action of GLP-1 is enhanced so that insulin release is promoted when food is eaten, the movement of food in the intestines is inhibited, and food intake and glucose release by the liver are reduced. The difference between DPP-4 inhibitors and GLP-1 analogues is that GLP-1 analogues are more potent (far more effective in lowering glucose levels and result in greater weight loss). Therefore, a person taking a GLP-1 analogue should not be taking a DPP-4 inhibitor as well.

Advantages

DPP-4 inhibitors are weight-neutral and have a low risk of hypoglycaemia, making them suitable for use in older adults, who may have some degree of renal failure and/or an increased risk of falls.

References

GPNotebookEducation (2020). What next after metformin in type 2 diabetes. https://gpnotebook.com/simplepage. cfm?ID=x2019062065928181497.

National Institute of Health and Care Excellence (2022). Type 2 Diabetes in Adults: Management. NICE Guideline NG28. Available at www.nice.org.uk/guidance/ng28.

Stewart, M. (2021). An overview of the oral medicines used in the management of type 2 diabetes. *Nurs. Stand.* 37 (1): 54–60. https://doi.org/10.7748/ns.2021.e11804.

Tahrani, A.A., Barnett, A.H., and Bailey, C.J. (2016). Pharmacology and therapeutic implications of current drugs for type 2 diabetes mellitus. *Nat. Rev. Endocrinol.* 12 (10): 566–592. https://doi. org/10.1038/nrendo.2016.86.

15 Insulin options

Figure 15.1 Insulin types.

Type of insulin	Examples	Onset of action	Peak	Duration	Comments
Rapid-acting	Apidra Humalog NovoRapid	5–15 minutes	30–60 minutes	2–5 hours	• Inject at the start of a meal
Short-acting	Actrapid	30 minutes	1–3 hours	Up to 8 hours	• Mainly used to make up IV insulin infusions in hospital
Intermediate-acting	Humulin I Insulatard Insuman basal	60–90 minutes	4–8 hours	12–14 hours	• Cloudy, so needs to be mixed before administration
Long-acting	Abasaglar Lantus Semglee Levemir	60–90 minutes	No peak	Up to 24 hours 18 hours	• Taken same time every day • Can be taken twice a day
Ultra-long acting	Tresiba	60–90 minutes	No peak	Up to 42 hours	• Once daily injection
Premixed/biphasic	Humalog Mix 25 Humalog Mix 50 Humulin M3 Insuman comb 50 Novomix 30	Biphasic onset: Short-acting/ rapid onset first, followed by Intermediate insulin	1–4 hours	12–14 hours	• Mealtime insulin • Cloudy, so needs to be mixed before administration

Five different types of insulin are used by people whose diabetes requires it. They all work differently, and some can be used in combination to suit the requirements of the individual. The different types of insulin, their onset of action, peak and duration are all charted in Figure 15.1. Different companies produce different brands of insulin, and these are listed in Figure 15.1 as well. The information detailed in the following sections comes from National Institute for Health and Care Excellence (2022) and Diabetes UK (2022).

Rapid-acting insulin

Rapid-acting insulin (also known as fast-acting insulin) is a mealtime insulin that starts working very quickly after injection. This insulin helps to manage the rise in glucose caused by eating carbohydrates in meals. It is taken just before starting to eat a meal as its onset of action is around 15 minutes. The insulin reaches its peak (maximum effectiveness) after about 90 minutes and its duration (time that it lasts for) is between two and five hours. This short duration is important: a person can have their three doses of rapid-acting insulin with their three meals if they are well spaced out. The colour of this insulin is clear, like water.

Short-acting insulin

Short-acting insulin is similar to rapid-acting insulin but works much slower. Before the newer rapid-acting insulins were available, this was the mealtime insulin. Short-acting insulin takes

about 30 minutes to start working, peaks after about two hours and can last in the body for up to eight hours. The eight-hour duration could be a problem if a person eats three meals a day because the doses would overlap and could cause hypoglycaemia. Thankfully, advances in science helped in developing rapid-acting insulin. Short-acting insulin is still being used in hospitals when nurses are giving an intravenous insulin infusion. The colour of this insulin is clear.

Long-acting insulin

Also known as background or basal insulin, this insulin works at a slow rate and is released into the body at a slow rate. After injection, the onset of action is about one hour; these insulins have no peak and the duration varies from 18 to 24 hours. There are some newer insulins called ultra-long-acting insulins and these can last up to 42 hours. These are mostly taken once a day, but some can be taken twice daily. People who are taking rapid-acting insulin at mealtimes will usually take a long-acting insulin to manage their blood glucose levels outside mealtimes, so they have 24-hour insulin cover. The colour of this insulin is clear.

Intermediate-acting insulins

These are also background insulins, because they have a long duration. Before long-acting insulins were developed, intermediate insulins were the only background insulins available. Their onset of action is also around one hour, they peak at about four to eight hours

Diabetes Care at a Glance, First Edition. Edited by Anne Phillips.
© 2023 John Wiley & Sons Ltd. Published 2023 by John Wiley & Sons Ltd.

after injection and their duration is around 12–14 hours. They therefore do not last 24 hours, and the peak presents a hypoglycaemia risk, particularly at night. People do still take this type of insulin as a background insulin or just on its own, to fit their requirements. The colour of this insulin is cloudy (similar to watered-down milk). Cloudy insulins need to be mixed before injection (Chapter 16 provides details of how to mix a cloudy insulin).

Premixed insulin

Also known as biphasic insulin, because it contains two types of insulin mixed together and the different insulins will start to work at different times or phases. It is a mixture of a short- or rapid-acting insulin and an intermediate-acting insulin. Thus instead of having two separate pens, premixed insulin comes in a two-in-one pen. Because it contains mealtime insulin, premixed insulin should be given at mealtimes. The insulin will have a number next to the name, for example 30 or 25. This number represents the percentage of rapid- or short-acting insulin in the mixture. The rest of it, 70 or 75%, comprises the intermediate-acting insulin. This insulin is cloudy and so needs to be mixed before injection.

References

Diabetes UK (2022). Insulin and diabetes. www.diabetes.org.uk/guide-to-diabetes/managing-your-diabetes/treating-your-diabetes/insulin (accessed 15 June 2022).

National Institute for Health and Care Excellence (2022). Treatment summaries: insulin. https://bnf.nice.org.uk/treatment-summaries/insulin (accessed 15 June 2022).

16 Insulin administration and injection technique

Figure 16.1 Injection sites.

Back of the Arms

Buttocks

Abdomen

Side of thighs

Figure 16.2 Correct and incorrect depth of injection needles.

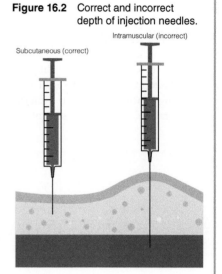

Subcutaneous (correct)

Intramuscular (incorrect)

Figure 16.3 Correct administration of an insulin injection using an injection pen. *Sources:* image 2, Alka5051/Adobe Stock; image 4, abidika/Adobe Stock; image 6, Remigiusz/Adobe Stock.

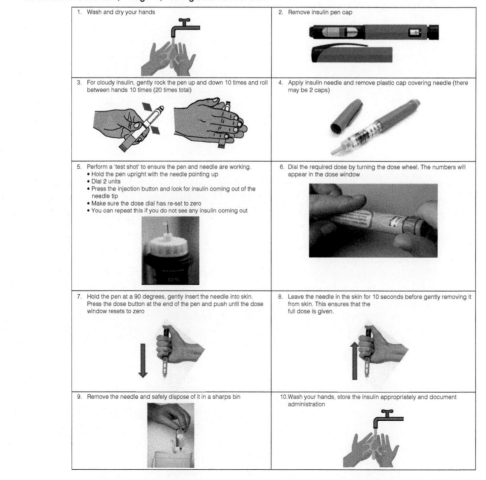

1. Wash and dry your hands

2. Remove insulin pen cap

3. For cloudy insulin, gently rock the pen up and down 10 times and roll between hands 10 times (20 times total)

4. Apply insulin needle and remove plastic cap covering needle (there may be 2 caps)

5. Perform a 'test shot' to ensure the pen and needle are working.
   - Hold the pen upright with the needle pointing up
   - Dial 2 units
   - Press the injection button and look for insulin coming out of the needle tip
   - Make sure the dose dial has re-set to zero
   - You can repeat this if you do not see any insulin coming out

6. Dial the required dose by turning the dose wheel. The numbers will appear in the dose window

7. Hold the pen at a 90 degrees, gently insert the needle into skin. Press the dose button at the end of the pen and push until the dose window resets to zero

8. Leave the needle in the skin for 10 seconds before gently removing it from skin. This ensures that the full dose is given.

9. Remove the needle and safely dispose of it in a sharps bin

10. Wash your hands, store the insulin appropriately and document administration

Diabetes Care at a Glance, First Edition. Edited by Anne Phillips.
© 2023 John Wiley & Sons Ltd. Published 2023 by John Wiley & Sons Ltd.

Figure 16.4 Correct performance of a skinfold. *Source:* Adapted from Trend Diabetes (2021).

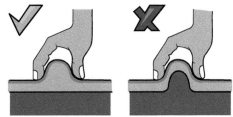

Figure 16.5 Layers of skin, fat and muscle (not to scale): the tip of a 4-mm needle will lie within the subcutaneous layer of fat.

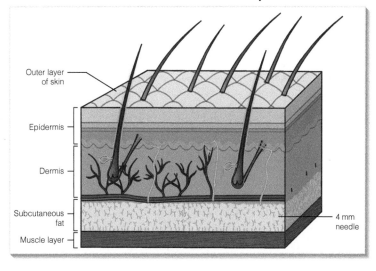

Insulin injection technique

Injection sites

There are several sites (areas) on the body where insulin can be injected. These areas contain a layer of fat just underneath the skin where the insulin is absorbed. Figure 16.1 shows the recommended injection sites: the abdomen, backs of arms, buttocks, and sides of the thighs. Injection into any other area carries a risk of injecting into sensitive nerves and larger blood vessels, which could result in pain or change in the rate of insulin absorption. Areas of skin with scar tissue or where the skin is broken should be avoided.

Figure 16.2 shows the correct and incorrect depth of injection.

How to give an injection using an insulin pen device

Figure 16.3 shows how to correctly administer an insulin injection using an injection pen (Trend Diabetes 2021). People who are very lean may need to inject into a skinfold, even with 4-mm needles. Figure 16.4 shows how to correctly perform a skinfold. The purpose of a skinfold is to lift the skin and fat away from the muscle to avoid injecting insulin into the muscle. The skin should be lifted using only the first two fingers and thumb, ensuring there is at least 1 cm between fingers and thumb. The skin should not be pinched as this might lift the muscle layer.

How deep to inject

Most insulin is available in the form of a pen device, and the needle sizes recommended are 4 or 5 mm. If the needle is too long, the insulin could be administered into the muscle. Figure 16.5 shows the layers of skin, fat and muscle (not to scale). The tip of a 4-mm needle in an average build person will lie within the subcutaneous layer of fat.

Injection needles

Whether using a pen or insulin syringe, the needle should never be reused as this could cause injection site problems and affect absorption of the insulin. Reusing the same needle not only presents an infection risk, but they bend, lose lubrication, and can cause damage and pain to the skin. Needles should always be disposed of in a sharps bin as soon as the injection is given.

Lipohypertrophy or lumps at the injection site

If the same small areas of skin are used many times, the fat tissue below the skin sometimes swells, a condition called lipohypertrophy (lipos). This creates large bumps that absorb insulin poorly. Too many injections into the same site may cause hard scar tissue to form under the skin, which also affects the body's ability to absorb insulin.

These bumps and scar tissue will usually disappear if the area is left alone for a while, usually two to three months. People who take insulin are encouraged to examine injection areas to help them select a site and prevent lumps or bumps. Healthcare professionals also need to ask people injecting insulin whether they can feel or see lipos, and when they see their patients face to face to always feel the injection sites for any lumps or hardness.

Site rotation

It is important to rotate injection sites to avoid lipohypertrophy and bruising. Ensure that injections are given in a different area at least 1 cm away from the last one.

Insulin storage

Insulin needs to be stored appropriately. Insulin that is not in use should be stored in a fridge at 2–8°C. The insulin that is in use can be stored at room temperature for up to 30 days. If stored in either excessively hot or excessively cold conditions, the insulin will become ineffective.

Reference

Trend Diabetes (2021). Injection technique matters: best practice in diabetes care. https://trenddiabetes.online/wp-content/uploads/2021/03/A5_Toolkit_2021_ITM_FINAL_v2.pdf (accessed 15 June 2022).

17 Insulin pump therapy

Figure 17.1 Insulin pump. *Source:* click_and_photo/Adobe Stock.　**Figure 17.2** Insulin pod. *Source:* Wavebreak Media/Adobe Stock.

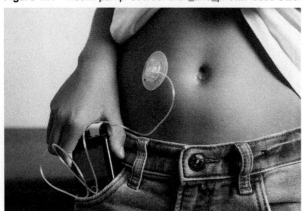

Figure 17.3 Infusion sites.

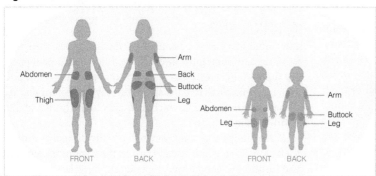

Figure 17.4 Basal-bolus insulin delivery.

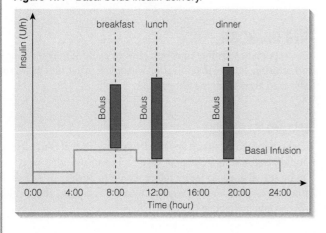

Table 17.1 Example of 24-hour basal rates.

Time	Basal Rate
0000	0.6 units/hour
01 00	0.6 units/hour
02:00	0.6 units/hour
0300	1.0 units/hour
0400	1.0 units/hour
0500	1.0 units/hour
0600	1.0 units/hour
0700	1.0 units/hour
0800	0.9 units/hour
0900	0.9 units/hour
1000	0.9 units/hour
1100	0.9 units/hour
1200	0.8 units/hour
1300	0.8 units/hour
1400	0.8 units/hour
1500	0.8 units/hour
1600	0.8 units/hour
1700	0.8 units/hour
1800	0.8 units/hour
1900	0.9 units/hour
2000	0.9 units/hour
2100	0.9 units/hour
2200	0.9 units/hour
2300	0.6 units/hour
20.2 units of basal insulin delivered over 24 hours	

Diabetes Care at a Glance, First Edition. Edited by Anne Phillips.
© 2023 John Wiley & Sons Ltd. Published 2023 by John Wiley & Sons Ltd.

Insulin pump therapy, also called continuous subcutaneous insulin infusion (CSII), is an alternative approach to delivering insulin. Instead of taking two to eight injections per day of two different types of long-acting and rapid-acting insulin, like someone on multiple daily injections, a person with diabetes wears a pocket-sized computerized pump. The pumps contain tiny motors that deliver insulin stored within a 200–300 unit reservoir inside the pump. A short length of tubing connects the pump to a small metal needle or plastic cannula that sits beneath the skin and enables insulin to be delivered into the subcutaneous tissue (Figure 17.1).

Pumps may have a small screen and buttons to enable the user to program and adjust how and when insulin is delivered. Alternatively, small disposable pumps called pods are worn by the person and a mobile phone-sized handset is used to program the pod (Figure 17.2).

The pump delivers one type of insulin: rapid-acting insulin. Rapid-acting insulin normally starts working within 10–20 minutes and reaches a peak of action between 60 and 90 minutes after it is injected. Rapid-acting insulin normally stops working approximately three to five hours after it has been injected.

Where the infusion set or pod is placed is called the infusion site. Common infusion sites for insulin pumps include the abdominal area, hips and bottom (Figure 17.3). People wearing pods may also use their upper arms. It is important that the infusion sites are changed and rotated every two to three days to ensure the skin remains healthy so that insulin can be absorbed and work as expected. Using the same site for more than three days increases the risks of infection in the short term and excess tissue growth (known as lipohypertrophy). Most people with diabetes using an insulin pump will reuse their infusion sites for more than 30 years so it is important that these sites remain healthy to ensure that insulin is quickly absorbed from the subcutaneous tissue at the infusion site.

The pump delivers this one type of insulin in two ways via the basal rate and a bolus (Figure 17.4). People wearing an insulin pump do not inject long-acting insulin. Instead, the basal rate acts like the background insulin in someone on multiple dose injection (MDI) therapy. It aims to maintain stable glucose levels. The pump constantly delivers very small amounts of rapid-acting insulin of 0.05 units. Table 17.1 shows the basal rate for a 24-hour period. The total amount of basal insulin is 20.2 units. This would be similar to someone on MDI taking one injection of 20 units of background insulin. However, for people wearing an insulin pump, the delivery of insulin is tailored to the individual, giving more or less insulin each hour. When set correctly, the basal rate should enable the person with diabetes to have stable glucose levels without eating or being active.

Pump users can also deliver a bolus of insulin when they eat a meal or to correct a high glucose value. At mealtimes, people with diabetes on MDI and insulin pumps are encouraged to match the amount of rapid-acting insulin to the amount of carbohydrates they eat at that meal. To do this, they use an insulin-to-carbohydrate ratio, for example 1 unit of insulin for every 10 g of carbohydrate that is eaten (Cheyette and Balolia 2016).

A meal bolus refers to the insulin the pump delivers at mealtimes to match the carbohydrate the person eats. For example, a person using an insulin pump would first estimate the amount of carbohydrate in their meal or snack, then enter the total grams of carbohydrate into their pump and the pump would calculate how much insulin to deliver based on the insulin-to-carbohydrate ratio programmed into the pump. Insulin can be delivered as a meal bolus whenever a person with diabetes eats a meal or a snack.

If a glucose level is above the person's target range four hours after they have eaten and taken insulin, they may choose to give insulin to lower their glucose. This correction bolus of insulin is intended to bring the high glucose reading back into the target range.

Troubleshooting high glucose readings

As insulin pumps only deliver rapid-acting insulin, the person with diabetes is at high risk of developing diabetic ketoacidosis (DKA) if the pump stops working or accidentally becomes disconnected (see Chapter 24 for more information on DKA). People using insulin pumps should always take action for any unexplained glucose levels above 14 mmol/l in order to prevent DKA:

- Check for ketones in the blood or urine.
- Take a correction bolus by injection instead of the pump.
- Change their infusion site and infusion set.
- Continue monitoring their glucose level until it returns to the target level.

Self-management guidance

People with diabetes who use insulin pumps are encouraged to follow these guidelines.

- Monitor glucose levels four or more times per day using continuous glucose monitoring (see Chapter 19) or blood glucose monitoring (see Chapter 18).
- Count carbohydrates: estimate carbohydrates in snacks and meals and give insulin each time food is eaten.
- Change the infusion site every two to three days.
- Carry a back-up insulin delivery system like a syringe or insulin pen in case the pump stops working.
- Work in partnership with the specialist diabetes team to adjust pump settings based on glucose levels.

Reference

Cheyette, C. and Balolia, Y. (2016). *Carbs & Cals: Carb and Calorie Counter*, 6e. UK: Chello Publishing.

18 # Self blood glucose monitoring

Figure 18.1 Blood-glucose monitoring procedure. *Sources:* Memorystockphoto / Adobe Stock; Oleksii Halutva / Adobe Stock; a.oleshko / Adobe Stock; megaflop / Adobe Stock; zothen / Adobe Stock; Elena Pimukova / Adobe Stock; Jakinnboaz / Adobe Stock; Onidji / Adobe Stock.

1. Wash your hands

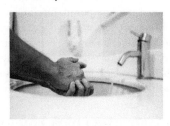

2. Ensure the person has washed their hands

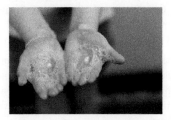

3. Switch on the glucometer and insert a new test strip

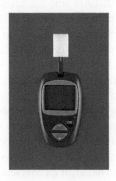

4. Wear Gloves and prick the side of the finger using a lancet

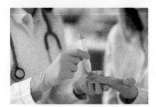

5. Touch the tip of the test strip against the blood droplet

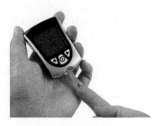

6. Apply pressure to the finger tip to stop the bleeding

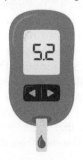

7. Record blood glucose result and report any unexpected reading

Wash Your Hands

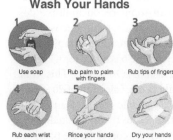

8. Wash hands and dispose of all PPE appropriately

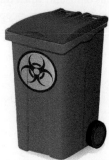

Diabetes Care at a Glance, First Edition. Edited by Anne Phillips.
© 2023 John Wiley & Sons Ltd. Published 2023 by John Wiley & Sons Ltd.

What is self blood glucose monitoring?

Self-monitoring of blood glucose refers to home blood glucose testing for people with diabetes. Self-monitoring is the use of regular blood testing to understand one's diabetes control and to inform changes that improve one's control or wider regime.

Benefits of blood glucose monitoring

Monitoring blood glucose (BG), also known as capillary blood glucose (CBG), levels shows the effect of a person's treatment and indicates if any changes in treatment are needed. Several clinical studies have revealed that maintaining good glycaemic control is critical in effectively managing diabetes, as well as reducing or preventing the various health complications associated with suboptimally controlled diabetes (glycaemic control refers to the typical levels of BG in a person with diabetes).

Who needs to monitor their blood glucose levels?

- People taking insulin.
- People on oral diabetes medication that may increase their risk of hypoglycaemia (including when driving or operating machinery).
- A person with diabetes who is pregnant or planning pregnancy.
- People on corticosteroids (e.g. prednisolone, hydrocortisone and dexamethasone). Steroids are discussed in Chapter 25.

Factors that influence BG levels

- Food: time of last food intake/quantity and type of carbohydrate consumed.
- Activity: timing in relation to food and medication and insulin doses, injection sites, type of exercise and BG level prior to starting exercise.
- Medications used for diabetes control and other medication such as steroids.
- Alcohol: type, food intake in relation to alcohol, amount of alcohol.
- Emotional well-being and stress.
- Kidney and liver function.
- Artificial feeding, for example total parenteral nutrition or via percutaneous endoscopic gastrostomy (PEG)/nasogastric (NG) tube.
- Obtaining the sample from unwashed hands.

When to monitor blood glucose

It is normal for BG levels to change throughout the day and for levels to rise after eating. The best times to test are just before a meal or two hours after a meal. This is because when BG levels rise due to eating, and a person takes their diabetes medication, it takes about two hours for their BG to return to pre-meal levels. Testing too soon after eating a meal or snack will likely register an elevated result. The frequency of testing will be determined by a number of factors and is decided by the person with diabetes in consultation with their healthcare professional.

The target range of BG levels is individualized for each person, in consultation with their diabetes healthcare professional. In addition to pre-meal testing, a person may need to perform a test at bedtime, particularly if they are taking diabetes treatment in the evening in order to reduce the risk of hypoglycaemia in the night (nocturnal hypoglycaemia).

When is BG monitoring unreliable?

The accuracy of CBG monitoring may be affected by clinical conditions, for example when a person has peripheral circulatory failure and severe dehydration, or in certain emergency situations when the body is trying to preserve blood flow to major organs and the blood supply to the fingers and toes (peripheries) can be severely reduced. This occurs in diabetes-related ketoacidosis (DKA), hyperosmolar hyperglycaemic state (HHS), hypotension and shock. These conditions cause peripheral shutdown, which can cause artificially low BG readings (DKA is covered in Chapter 24). In this case, a blood sample taken from a vein may provide a more reliable BG result.

How to self-monitor blood glucose

Self-monitoring of blood glucose is performed on capillary blood samples generally obtained from pricking the side of the finger, although alternative sites may be used. Blood in the finger responds rapidly to changes in BG. However, fingertips contain nerve endings and can become sore and less sensitive with frequent testing and it is therefore important to sample from different fingers. It is advisable to avoid the forefinger and thumb, as they are used more frequently throughout the day.

The process of CBG monitoring (Figure 18.1) (Diabetes UK 2017)

Gather the relevant equipment

- Glucometer (perform a control test first if required)
- Single-use safety lancets
- Testing strips: make sure the expiry date is valid
- Gauze
- Sharps bin

Procedure

- Ensure person's hands are washed with soap and water (do not use alcohol gel/wipes on the hands as this could affect result; alcohol wipes also harden the skin).
- Ensure meter is switched on and insert test strip.
- Lance a finger with the device.
- Apply blood droplet to test strip according to manufacturer's instructions.
- Place gauze over puncture site, apply firm pressure and monitor for excess bleeding.
- Dispose of lancet and gloves appropriately, and wash hands.
- Document the BG reading.

Advances in BG monitoring

A variety of devices is available for people with diabetes to monitor their glucose levels, including flash and continuous glucose monitoring (discussed in Chapter 19). In an inpatient setting, it is still recommended that CBG monitoring uses an approved quality-assured meter.

Reference

Diabetes UK (2017) Self-monitoring of blood glucose levels for adults with type 2 diabetes (March 2017). Available at www.diabetes.org.uk/professionals/position-statements-reports/diagnosis-ongoing-management-monitoring/self-monitoring-of-blood-glucose-levels-for-adults-with-type-2-diabetes

19 Continuous and flash glucose monitoring

Figure 19.1 Intermittently scanned glucose sensor: Freestyle Libre 2. *Source:* Abbott.

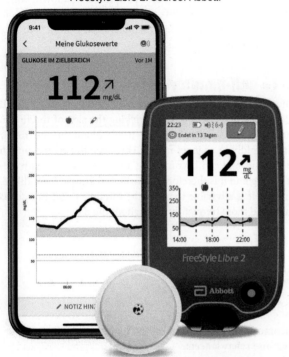

Table 19.1 Trend arrows[a].

Trend arrow	Rate and direction of glucose change	Anticipated change in glucose from current reading	
		15 min	30 min
↑	Glucose rising rapidly >0.1 mmol/l/min	>+1.5 mmol/l	>+3.0 mmol/l
↗	Glucose rising 0.06–0.1 mmol/l/min	0.9 to 1.5 mmol/l	1.8 to 3.0 mmol/l
→	Glucose changing slowly <0.06 mmol/l/min	< ± 0.9 mmol/l	< ± 1.8 mmol/l
↘	Glucose falling 0.06–0.1 mmol/l/min	−0.9 to −1.5 mmol/l	−1.8 to −3.0 mmol/l
↓	Glucose falling rapidly >0.1 mmol/l/min	>−1.5 mmol/l	>-3.0 mmol/l

[a] Note that trend arrows are not always concurrent with a laboratory reference measurement of blood glucose change when measured at the same time.

Figure 19.2 Sensor locations.

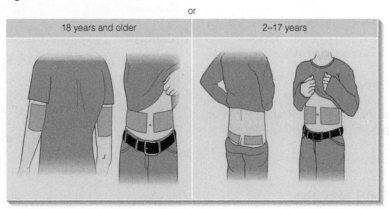

Figure 19.3 Glucose in the interstitial blood is measured.

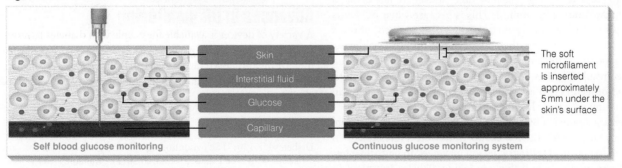

Diabetes Care at a Glance, First Edition. Edited by Anne Phillips.
© 2023 John Wiley & Sons Ltd. Published 2023 by John Wiley & Sons Ltd.

In order for people with diabetes and their healthcare professionals to successfully manage diabetes, they need to know the person's glucose levels. Traditionally, glucose has been measured using a small drop of blood obtained from the finger (see Chapter 18). New glucose sensing technologies now provide alternatives to measuring blood glucose.

Key components of continuous glucose monitoring (CGM) systems include a glucose sensor, a transmitter, a glucose reader and software for accessing glucose reports. This chapter discusses the glucose sensor, transmitter, reader and basic glucose data. Chapter 20 examines the software and reports used to analyze and interpret the glucose data.

All people with type 1 diabetes in the UK, people with type 2 diabetes on multiple daily injections, pregnant women and people with learning difficulties and diabetes can be funded to use intermittently scanned glucose sensing (isCGM) or real-time glucose sensing (rtCGM). Some people may also self-fund these technologies.

CGM systems continuously measure glucose through a small sensor that is inserted underneath the skin. A small adhesive patch holds the sensor in place along with a transmitter and battery that sit above the skin encased in plastic (Figure 19.1). Each sensor can be worn for between 7 and 14 days depending on the brand. Sensors can be worn in different locations (Figure 19.2). When a sensor stops working, it is removed and a new sensor is inserted.

Rather than directly measuring blood glucose, the sensor indirectly measures glucose in the interstitial fluid – the fluid surrounding the layers of the skin – by detecting electrical signals (Figure 19.3). These signals are collected and converted using algorithms. New glucose readings are displayed every one to five minutes either on a hand-held reader or a smartphone app using the same units as those used for blood glucose monitoring (e.g. mmol/l). Differences between interstitial CGM readings and blood glucose readings are normally parallel, although there is a five-minute time delay between CGM and blood glucose readings due to the way it is measured and where the glucose is within the body. Additionally, there can be differences in both when glucose values are changing rapidly.

Collected glucose data can be displayed as reports on the handsets or software management system and analyzed by people with diabetes and their healthcare providers to adjust insulin delivery and inform diabetes self-management (see Chapter 20). In addition to the glucose value, CGM readings also display a trend arrow that indicates whether the glucose is rising, stable or falling, along with how quickly the change is occurring (Table 19.1). Trend arrows and glucose values combine to help people with diabetes to predict what their glucose levels will soon be and inform their self-management decisions.

Consider this example: Sabine is a 26-year-old woman with type 1 diabetes. She is about to drive her car to the supermarket with her one-year-old son. If she were to test her blood glucose and see a reading of 7 mmol/l, she would likely feel that she would be safe to drive her car. However, if she was wearing CGM and saw the same value of 7 mmol/l along with a trend arrow pointing down, this would indicate that her glucose level is falling rapidly. To avoid experiencing low glucose while driving or shopping, Sabine may decide to take some fast-acting glucose and delay her trip until her CGM displays a flat arrow, indicating that her glucose is stable, or an upward arrow, indicating that her glucose is rising.

There are currently two categories of CGM: rtCGM and isCGM, also known as flash glucose monitoring. rtCGM was the first type of CGM to be developed, around 2002. rtCGM automatically displays the glucose data on the reader and app; it also sounds an alert warning the user when the glucose level is predicted to go above or below their target range and when the glucose value moves outside the specified range. These alerts and alarms can enable the person with diabetes or their carers to take pre-emptive action, such as drinking some juice before they experience low glucose. These alerts and alarms are especially helpful for people with hypoglycaemic unawareness, for those who experience any symptoms of low blood glucose (see Chapter 22), for those who are tightly controlling their glucose levels like pregnant women with diabetes, or for those who may need someone else to take action (e.g. young children). rtCGM is an important part of automated insulin delivery (AID) systems. rtCGM supplies glucose data to an app that automatically changes the insulin delivery in an insulin pump with the aim of maintaining the glucose within a target range. These systems are becoming more widely available for people with type 1 diabetes.

isCGM was released in 2017 and is known as the Freestyle Libre glucose sensor; it measures interstitial glucose. However, unlike rtCGM, the glucose data and trend arrow are only displayed when the user scans the sensor with a hand-held reader or mobile phone app. Due in part to its lower cost, flash glucose monitoring became widely available on prescription as an alternative to self-blood glucose monitoring. Libre 2 was later released, which alerted the user to scan when the glucose values were outside the target range. isCGM has since become synonymous with flash glucose monitoring.

Some people may develop allergic skin reactions to the adhesives used in some of the sensors. Symptoms can range from relatively mild, such as minimal redness and inflammation, to moderate itching and severe sloughing of the skin. Protective barriers and sprays may help to diminish these reactions. Alternatively, some individuals may need to change to a different type of CGM or stop using CGM altogether.

Alerts and alarms can be useful features. However, they can also become frustrating if they occur frequently. People with diabetes need to understand that these alarms could potentially cause disruption and draw attention to themselves. Plans need to be made for avoiding alerts and alarms sounding at inappropriate times.

Overall, CGM benefits people with diabetes by providing clear insights into their glucose values.

Interpreting glucose data

Figure 20.1 Haemogloblin A1c (HbA1c).

Red Blood Cells
Glucose
HbA1c

Figure 20.2 CGM report summary page.

Glucose		
Average Glucose	Time in Range	Sensor Usage
8.4 mmol/L	0% Very high	Days with CGM Data
	31% high	86%
	68% Mid Range	6/7
	1% Low	
	0% Very Low	
Standard Deviation GMI	Target Range:	Avg. calibrations er day
2.1 mmol/L N/A	Day (06:00–22:00): 3.9–10.0 mmol/L	86%
	Night (22:00–06:00): 4.4–8.3 mmol/L	

Figure 20.3 Time in range.

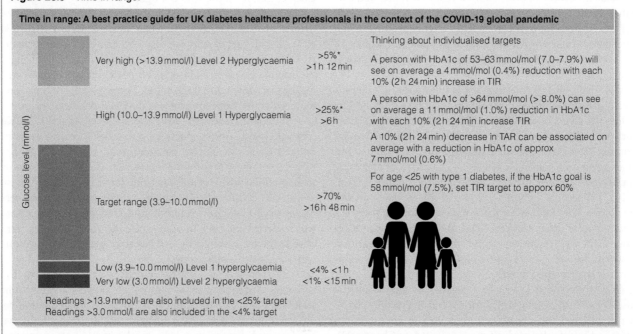

Time in range: A best practice guide for UK diabetes healthcare professionals in the context of the COVID-19 global pandemic

Glucose level (mmol/l)

Very high (>13.9 mmol/l) Level 2 Hyperglycaemia — >5%* / >1 h 12 min

High (10.0–13.9 mmol/l) Level 1 Hyperglycaemia — >25%* / >6 h

Target range (3.9–10.0 mmol/l) — >70% / >16 h 48 min

Low (3.9–10.0 mmol/l) Level 1 hyperglycaemia — <4% <1 h
Very low (3.0 mmol/l) Level 2 hyperglycaemia — <1% <15 min

Readings >13.9 mmol/l are also included in the <25% target
Readings >3.0 mmol/l are also included in the <4% target

Thinking about individualised targets

A person with HbA1c of 53–63 mmol/mol (7.0–7.9%) will see on average a 4 mmol/mol (0.4%) reduction with each 10% (2 h 24 min) increase in TIR

A person with HbA1c of >64 mmol/mol (> 8.0%) can see on average a 11 mmol/mol (1.0%) reduction in HbA1c with each 10% (2 h 24 min increase TIR

A 10% (2 h 24 min) decrease in TAR can be associated on average with a reduction in HbA1c of approx 7 mmol/mol (0.6%)

For age <25 with type 1 diabetes, if the HbA1c goal is 58 mmol/mol (7.5%), set TIR target to apporx 60%

Figure 20.4 CGM daily report.

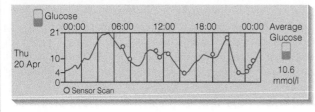

Table 20.1 HbA1c and average blood glucose values.

HbA1c mmol/mol (IFCC)	HbA1c % (DCCT)	Estimated average blood glucose (mmol/l)
42	6	6.9
53	7	8.5
64	8	10.2
75	9	11.8
86	10	13.3
97	11	14.9
108	12	16.5
119	13	18.1

Understanding glucose data is key to supporting people with diabetes. This chapter explores three different forms of glucose data: haemoglobin A1c (HbA1c), blood glucose records, and continuous glucose monitoring (CGM) reports.

HbA1c

HbA1c is a blood test that measures how much glucose is attached to a red blood cell (Figure 20.1). It provides an average of an individual's blood glucose for the previous three months (Table 20.1). HbA1c is an important indicator that reflects the risk a person with diabetes has of developing long-term complications such as blindness, kidney failure or nerve damage.

HbA1c is used in clinics to provide a target reading. For example, the National Institute for Health and Care Excellence (NICE) recommends that adults with type 1 diabetes aim for a target HbA1c of 48 mmol/mol (6.5%) or lower, again to minimize the risk of developing diabetes-related complications. Less than 10% of people living with type 1 diabetes in the UK achieve this target. Over 70% have HbA1c values greater than or equal to 58 mmol/mol (7.5%) and over 40% have greater than 70 mmol/mol (8.6%). Many people with diabetes remain at high risk of developing diabetes-related complications.

HbA1c is widely used to provide an overview of someone's diabetes control. However, it lacks important details, such as how often the individual experiences high and low blood glucose levels, that help to guide self-management.

Blood glucose records

Most people with diabetes monitor their blood glucose readings and are encouraged to record these readings in diaries or logbooks (see Chapter 18). These records provide snapshots of what the glucose levels were at specific points throughout the day. If the person also recorded the times that they ate meals and took medication (e.g. the time, type and amount of insulin), knowledgeable healthcare professionals could adjust the medication to enable glucose values to reflect the recommended blood glucose target ranges. Glucose monitoring is widely used for diabetes care.

Continuous glucose monitoring reports

With the increasing use of CGM, new ways of viewing glucose data have arisen. This is due in part to the large amount of data that is collected. When a person with diabetes tests blood glucose, there are gaps in the day between the tests. CGM fills in these gaps so that people with diabetes and their healthcare professionals can see how the glucose changes minute by minute throughout the day and also provides averages over a week or longer. This makes it easier to identify what may be causing the glucose to rise or fall and to explore options to address any undesired changes.

Analyzing glucose data

Glucose data can be viewed in various ways. The following provides some examples and advice for interpreting the information presented on CGM reports.

A summary page provides an overview of glucose data (Figure 20.2). This report can be read from right to left. First, look at the sensor usage (A), which provides information about how much data has been collected over a specific time frame. This example shows 86% of data captured. If sensor usage is greater than 80%, the rest of the data provided should be trustworthy. For sensor usage less than 80%, it may be worthwhile looking at other reports. Average calibrations per day (B) provides the number of blood glucose tests used to calibrate the CGM sensor. Some sensors require one or more calibrations per day while others do not require any calibrations.

Time in range (C) provides a breakdown of the glucose sensor values by time in range (TIR), time below range (TBR) and time above range (TAR). International time-in-range guidelines developed in 2019 recommend various ranges for children and adults with type 1 and type 2 diabetes, pregnant women and frail populations (Figure 20.3). The specific target ranges in this example are 3.9–10 mmol/l from 0600 to 2200 and 4.4–8.3 mmol/l from 2200 to 0600. TIR is 68% and TBR is 1% so concerns about hypoglycaemia are unlikely. A TAR of 31% is acceptable so changes to this person's diabetes management would be minimal. This is supported by the average glucose (D) and the glucose management indicator (GMI) (E), which provides an estimated HbA1c value based on this glucose data.

Daily glucose values from CGM can also be viewed over 24-hour periods (Figure 20.4). The readings start at midnight, with each vertical line representing a two-hour time block (e.g. 0000–0200, 0200–0400, 0400–0600, etc.), and run until midnight. The glucose values are displayed on the left vertical axis. The target range is between 4 and 10 mmol/l and the range is 0–20 mmol/l. This 24-hour trace shows the glucose values rising from 0200 to 0600 and then dropping until 0900 and subsequently rising before falling just after 1200. These data help to identify daily profiles and can be viewed over multiple days to identify patterns. This can help to guide treatment decisions like insulin dosages.

Most people with diabetes do not use CGM and therefore management decisions will still be made using HbA1c and blood glucose logbooks.

21 Blood pressure and lipid management

Figure 21.1 Identifying cardiovascular risk.

Assess cardiovascular risk factors annually:
1. Estimated glomerular filtration rate (eGFR) and urine albumin/creatinine ratio (ACR)
2. Smoking status
3. Blood glucose control
4. Blood pressure
5. Full lipid profile, including high-density lipoprotein (HDL) and low-density lipoprotein (LDL), cholesterol and triglycerides
6. Age
7. Family history of cardiovascular disease
8. Abdominal adiposity

Figure 21.3 Aims for cholesterol levels in people with diabetes.

A Cholesterol test can measure:
- Total cholesterol: the amount of cholesterol in the blood (including good and bad cholesterol)
- HDL (called good cholesterol): this reduces the risk of heart attacks and strokes
- LDL and non-HDL cholesterol – this increases the risk of heart attacks and strokes
- Triglycerides – a fatty substance similar to LDL

Levels (mmol/l) to aim for:

Total cholesterol	4 or below
HDL (good cholesterol)	1 or above
LDL (bad cholesterol)	3 or below
Non-HDL (bad cholesterol)	4 or below
Triglycerides	2.3 or below

Figure 21.2 Why we control blood pressure.

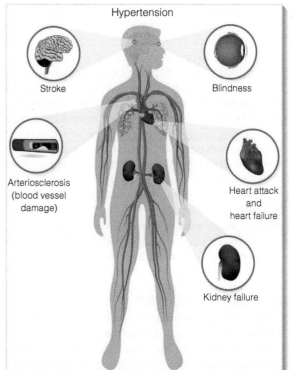

Figure 21.4 Stages of atherosclerosis.

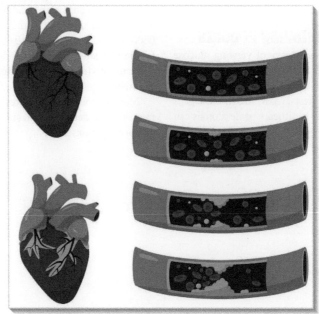

Diabetes Care at a Glance, First Edition. Edited by Anne Phillips.
© 2023 John Wiley & Sons Ltd. Published 2023 by John Wiley & Sons Ltd.

In people with type 2 diabetes the overall risk of cardiovascular disease, which includes myocardial infarction (heart attacks) and cerebrovascular accidents (strokes), is more than double that of the general population. Blood pressure and lipid management is pivotal for people with type 1 and type 2 diabetes in order to reduce their cardiovascular risk (Figure 21.1).

The World Health Organization (2021) identified that hypertension (high blood pressure) is a serious medical condition that significantly increases the risk of heart, brain, kidney and other disease. Regular monitoring of blood pressure is very important, and the National Institute for Health and Care Excellence (NICE) clinical guidelines (2022a) recommends that all people with type 2 diabetes have a target blood pressure of less than 140/80 mmHg or less than 130/80 mmHg in people with kidney, eye or cerebrovascular damage. When managing blood pressure in people with type 2 diabetes, lifestyle factors (smoking status, alcohol intake, obesity, and lack of exercise) should be discussed and appropriate support offered to each individual in a person-centred way. In people with type 2 diabetes, NICE (2019) recommends measuring standing as well as sitting blood pressure to monitor for postural hypotension.

Obesity is associated with increased blood pressure and people should be encouraged to achieve their ideal body weight, to reduce dietary salt intake and to undertake regular aerobic exercise. In people with chronic kidney disease and/or positive microalbuminuria, the blood pressure target is lowered in order to reduce pressure on the renal system and earlier introduction of antihypertensive agents is advised.

In people with type 1 diabetes with blood pressure at or above 135/85 mmHg (or 130/80 mmHg with high arterial risk), NICE (2022b) recommends commencing antihypertensive treatments. The person needs to be enabled to make an informed decision about the choice of agent by considering individual factors and the risk of pregnancy. NICE (2022a) recommends titrating antihypertensives in a stepwise fashion in order to reach the blood pressure targets recommended and to monitor blood pressure annually in the surgery and to promote home blood pressure monitoring on calibrated equipment. Multiple medications will often be required to achieve adequate control of hypertension and individuals need to be asked about potential side effects such as a dry cough with angiotensin-converting enzyme (ACE) inhibitors, lethargy, postural hypotension and sexual dysfunction.

Controlling blood pressure is an optimum aim is cardiovascular risk reduction (Figure 21.2).

Annual assessment of cardiovascular risk in people with diabetes should include a full lipid profile. If the individual has a history of high triglyceride levels, then a fasting lipid profile is recommended (NICE 2022b). If a fasting sample is required, advise the individual to take their insulin or oral antihyperglycaemic agents after the sample has been taken in order to avoid post-meal hypoglycaemia. In diabetes care, the target for lipid levels is 4 mmol/l, which is lower than that for the population without diabetes. Cholesterol is measured in three ways and the aim of treatment is to reduce the total cholesterol level and to increase the high-density lipoprotein (HDL) cholesterol level (Figure 21.3).

Statin therapies work directly on the liver by inhibiting hydroxymethylglutaryl coenzyme A (HMG-CoA) reductase, an enzyme that is involved in the early stages of cholesterol synthesis in the liver. Statins also promote the removal of low-density and very low-density lipoproteins from the blood. Statins are generally well tolerated, but some people can experience general muscular aching and if this occurs changing the brand of statin can help. Treating lipids can help reduce atherosclerosis (thickening or hardening of the arteries by plaques made from fatty substances and cholesterol) and this is important in order to reduce the risk of myocardial infarction and peripheral vascular disease (Figure 21.4).

We therefore encourage people to self-monitor their blood pressure at home and report their findings to keep regular checks on treatment escalation and adjustment needs.

References

National Institute for Health and Care Excellence (2019). Hypertension in Adults: Diagnosis and Management. NICE Guideline NG136. www.nice.org.uk/guidance/ng136.

National Institute for Health and Care Excellence (2022a). Type 2 Diabetes in Adults: Management. NICE Guideline NG28. www.nice.org.uk/guidance/ng28.

National Institute for Health and Care Excellence (2022b). Type 1 Diabetes in Adults: Diagnosis and Management. NICE Guideline NG17. www.nice.org.uk/guidance/ng17.

World Health Organization (2021). Guideline for the Pharmacological Treatment of Hypertension in Adults. https://apps.who.int/iris/rest/bitstreams/1365359/retrieve.

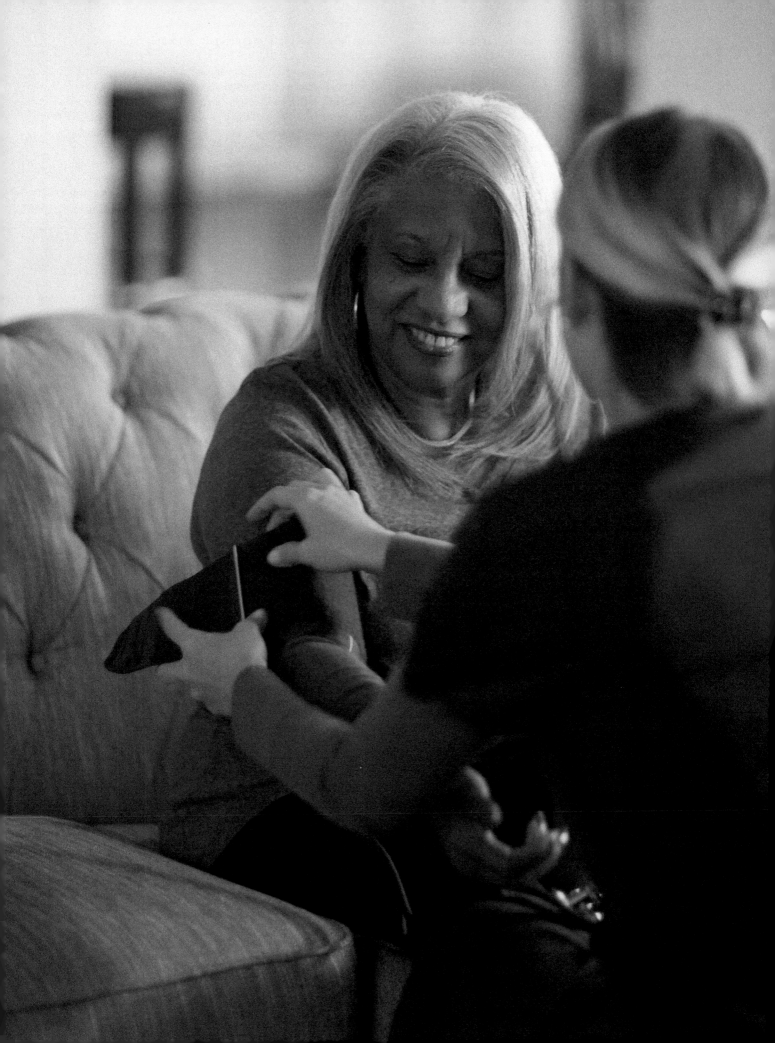

Acute complications

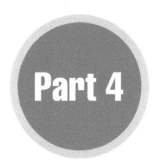

Part 4

Chapters

22 Recognizing and treating hypoglycaemia

Figure 22.1 Factors which affect blood glucose levels during the day and night.

- Type of food consumed
- Timing of medication and meals
- Physical activity
- Medications
- Age
- Stress
- Dehydration
- Temperature in the environment
- Illness
- Menstrual periods
- Alcohol
- Renal function

Figure 22.2 Symptoms of hypoglycaemia.

- Lightheadedness
- Dizziness
- Confusion
- Irritability
- Lack of concentration
- Nervousness
- Shakiness
- Anxiety
- Pallor
- Sweating
- Clamminess
- Palpitations and a fast heart rate
- Hunger
- Sleepiness
- Fainting
- Tingling lips and tongue
- Or no symptoms at all to the individual if they have hypo unawareness

Figure 22.3 Progress of hypoglycaemia.

Diabetes Care at a Glance, First Edition. Edited by Anne Phillips.

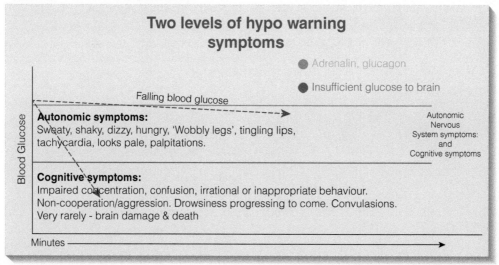

This chapter is to help you understand what hypoglycaemia is but also to help you treat hypoglycaemia effectively. The Hypobox, which is available in many NHS trusts, GP practices and schools, is a an important tool to help people who may be potentially or actually experiencing low blood glucose (known as hypoglycaemia) and who may need your help.

Someone with either type 1 or type 2 diabetes treated with glucose-lowering medications (e.g. insulin or sulfonylureas such as gliclazide) can experience low blood glucose or hypoglycaemia. The usual blood glucose levels for people without diabetes range from 3.5 to 6.5 mmol/l (63–117 mg/dl). Blood glucose varies with food intake and measurements are usually taken before eating (preprandial) and after eating (postprandial). For people with diabetes the aim is for the lowest blood glucose to be 4 mmol/l (72 mg/dl) and to treat with fast-acting glucose if the blood glucose is below 4 mmol/l. This is commonly known as '4 is the floor'. Various factors affect blood glucose levels and these are listed in Figure 22.1.

The brain is dependent on glucose to function effectively. Because the brain cannot store glucose, it needs a constant supply; consequently, as blood glucose levels start to fall, the brain is unable to function as normal, a condition known as neuroglycopenia. If blood glucose starts to fall below 4 mmol/l (72 mg/dl), then the individual begins to experience different signs and symptoms and their behaviour may change (Figures 22.2 and 22.3). Initially the individuals affected may appear confused, flustered or quite disorientated and may not recognize these symptoms themselves.

Affected individuals will also develop pallor, but sometimes a bluish tinge appears around their lips and tongue. They will also start to sweat very suddenly and profusely, called a cold sweat; this is different from the normal sweating that occurs after physical activity or exercise. Individuals may start shaking and lack coordination so that they are unable to carry out your instructions or requests for them to sit down; if this occurs, you will be required to guide them to a place of safety.

The lack of glucose also causes an increase in heart rate and individuals can experience palpitations and consequent release of adrenaline, which in some people may induce anxiety, discomfort and fear. As the blood glucose drops even further, individuals start to become sleepy. Not everybody will exhibit the signs and symptoms in the same way, as it depends on the individual and also on how rapidly the blood glucose is falling.

It is important to remember that these signs and symptoms are simply indications of what people might present with and that hypoglycaemia is only one cause. If the individual's signs and symptoms cannot differentiate between hypoglycaemia and hyperglycaemia, start treatment for low blood glucose because it is very important to avoid the risk of fitting (seizures).

In the first instance, individuals should be encouraged to treat themselves and hopefully they will have some fast-acting glucose stores on their person. However, low blood glucose causes some people's characters to change completely, and they can become very aggressive, very vocal, or may cry. This is worth bearing in mind especially with those who have lived with diabetes a long time and have avoided taking fast-acting glucose, so may resist attempts to give glucose to them.

It is recommended to use pure glucose sources first, for example dextrose tablets or a glucose-type drink. The reason for this is because pure glucose is rapidly absorbed and released into the bloodstream to increase blood glucose. Combinations of glucose and fructose (a fruit sugar found in smooth orange juice, jelly beans or small bags of sweets) are absorbed slower. If this is the only option available, then it should be used, but try to treat with the quickest option first.

Avoid using anything containing chocolate, for example a chocolate bar or a chocolate bar with toffee, because they contain a lot of fat and fat is very slow to be absorbed, so is not a good treatment for hypoglycaemia. In particular, avoid hot drinks containing sugar because there is a risk of burns if they are spilt.

The person should recover within about 5–10 minutes. Once recovery occurs and the blood glucose level has returned to above 4 mmol/l (72 mg/dl), encourage the individual to eat some carbohydrate-rich food, for example a sandwich or a banana or a couple of biscuits. Reassure them that they are recovering because they will be very frightened and potentially a bit embarrassed about what has happened.

If recovery has not occurred and the blood glucose is still less than 4 mmol/l (72 mg/dl) after 5–10 minutes, then repeat the treatment and try to use a quick-acting glucose store. However, if recovery has still not occurred after the repeat treatment, and the individual is becoming unconscious or fitting, then help is required immediately. Place the person in the recovery position and ring the resus bell in hospital or call 999 in the community.

Any intervention is for the individual's own safety and so the most important aims are to treat the hypoglycaemia, treat the low blood glucose, enable the person to recover, and then follow up with a carbohydrate source of food. Document the hypoglycaemia and seek medical or diabetes specialist nursing review.

23 Sick day advice

Figure 23.1 Sick day management advice for type 1 diabetes. *Source:* Adapted from Down (2020), Diabetes UK (2020) and Trend UK (2020a).

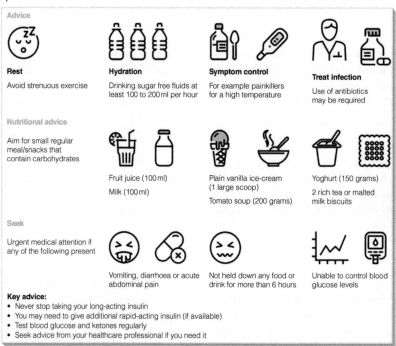

Figure 23.2 Sick day management advice for type 2 diabetes. *Source:* Adapted from Down (2020), Diabetes UK (2020) and Trend UK (2020b).

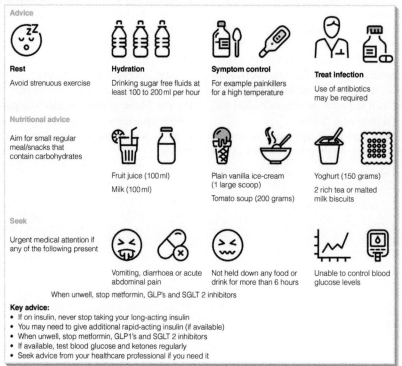

Like most people, those living with diabetes occasionally experience intercurrent illness, which has the potential to cause acute complications. Any intercurrent illness can cause glucose levels to rise and these include the common cold, diarrhoea and vomiting, and urinary tract infections. Intercurrent illness is the development of a new disease or illness occurring during the progress of another condition.

The recent COVID-19 outbreak has added to the list of illnesses and the need to reiterate self-management advice to people living with diabetes. Recent studies have linked an increased prevalence and poor outcomes with COVID-19 in people with both type 1 and type 2 diabetes. If blood glucose levels are not well controlled before hospital admission, people with diabetes and COVID-19 generally take longer to recover or have long-term effects from the condition.

How illness affects management of diabetes

The stress response due to illness results in the body preparing itself by ensuring that energy (glucose) is readily available. Insulin levels fall and hyperglycaemia results from the release of stress hormones such as glucagon and adrenaline (epinephrine), which oppose the action of insulin. The action of glucagon leads to increased glucose release by the liver and a rise in growth hormone and cortisol levels, causing body tissues (muscle and fat) to become less sensitive to insulin (called insulin resistance). As a result, more glucose is present in the bloodstream and although the individual may not have missed their dose of medication, the effect of illness increases their insulin requirements. Previous chapters have shown that insulin is required by the body to move excess glucose from the bloodstream to the cells that need glucose for energy. Ketones are formed by the liver as an alternative source of energy when the cells cannot access the glucose because of a shortage of insulin (see Chapter 24).

The symptoms that a person can experience when unwell are:

- feeling thirstier than usual
- feeling nauseated or vomiting
- elevated glucose levels
- elevated ketone levels
- passing more urine than usual.
- Urgent medical attention should be sought if the individual is drowsy or is vomiting or is experiencing abdominal pain and fast deep breathing as these are very serious symptoms.

Acute complications

People living with diabetes may be able to self-manage hyperglycaemia and a minor degree of ketonaemia; however, there is always a risk of developing acute complications such as diabetic ketoacidosis (DKA) and hyperosmolar hyperglycaemic state (HHS). Occasional hyperglycaemia (elevated blood glucose levels) is a common occurrence in both type 1 and type 2 diabetes and is usually resolved by adjusting either carbohydrate intake or insulin dosage.

However, if diabetes is not managed well during illness it can escalate and result in more serious conditions such as DKA and HHS, which would require emergency hospital admission. DKA and HHS are discussed in Chapter 24.

What people need to know when managing their diabetes during illness

People living with diabetes need to know how to manage blood glucose during periods of illness (called sick-day management). This includes specific information about frequency of blood glucose monitoring, blood glucose targets, checking for ketones, what ketone testing results in urine or blood indicate, taking extra quick-acting insulin, appropriate adjustment of insulin doses, identifying early signs and symptoms of DKA or HHS, and knowing when to contact the diabetes specialist team. Additionally, advice should be given about what medications should be stopped in episodes of vomiting and diarrhoea and when to escalate their care accordingly.

People with diabetes need to have adequate access to repeat prescriptions of the equipment that will enable them to manage their condition during illness. This includes glucose strips, ketone testing strips, and lancets for those who usually use them (mainly people taking insulin or diabetes medication that can cause hypoglycaemia or who are pregnant).

Organizations such as Trend Diabetes UK have produced handy, easy-to-follow leaflets regarding sick-day management for individuals with type 1 and 2 diabetes that healthcare practitioners can not only use themselves, but signpost to people with diabetes.

Figures 23.1 and 23.2 summarize the sick day management advice for people living with diabetes.

Summary

Whilst most people living with diabetes are successfully self-managing when they are well, illness can have a variety of effects on a person's glycaemic control and overall well-being. The overall effect of illness could result in temporary erratic glucose levels but could also lead to serious complications such as DKA and HHS.

References

Diabetes UK(2020). Diabetes when you're unwell. www.diabetes.org.uk/guide-to-diabetes/life-with-diabetes/illness (accessed 1 July 2022).

Down, S. (2020). How to advise on sick day rules. *Diabet. Prim. Care* 22(3): 47–48. https://diabetesonthenet.com/wp-content/uploads/pdf/dotn024ae8fb1b78500b7bc752b98e9b6d92.pdf (accessed 1 July 2022).

Trend UK (2020a). Type 1 diabetes: what to do when you are ill. https://trenddiabetes.online/wp-content/uploads/2020/03/A5_T1Illness_TREND_FINAL.pdf (accessed 1 July 2022).

Trend UK (2020b). Type 2 diabetes: what to do when you are Ill. https://trenddiabetes.online/wp-content/uploads/2020/03/A5_T2Illness_TREND_FINAL.pdf (accessed 1 July 2022).

24 Diabetes-related ketoacidosis

Figure 24.1 Comparison between DKA and HHS.

- Signs and symptoms of DKA:

Remember...

- Signs and symptoms of DKA often develop quickly, sometimes within 24 hours

- DKA is potentially life-threatening and requires urgent hospital admission

- Signs and symptoms of HHS:

Remember...

- HHS occurs gradually over a few days

- Can overlap with symptoms of DKA

- HHS is potentially life-threatening and requires urgent hospital admission

• Polydipsia (excessive thirst)	• Elevated blood glucose levels of above 30 mmol/l
• Polyuria (excessive or an abnormally large production of urine)	• Confusion – new confusion or worsening of pre-existing confusion
• Dehydration (dry mouth, tongue, skin)	• Polyuria
• Laboured breathing	• Polydipsia
• Abdominal pain	• Dehydration
• Nausea and vomiting	• Nausea
• Drowsiness	• Gradual drowsiness
• Confusion	• Loss of consciousness
• The smell of ketones on breath (pear-drops)	
• Ketones in urine dipstick or blood ketone test	

Diabetes-related ketoacidosis (DKA) is a potentially life-threatening condition when there is severe lack of insulin. This means the body's cells cannot access glucose for energy and start to use fat instead. The liver breaks down fats, and compounds called ketones are produced by this process. When ketones are released, they can be a useful source of energy in emergency situations. However, if left unchecked, ketones can accumulate and make blood acidic, hence the term 'acidosis' (JBDS-IP 2021).

Who can develop it?

DKA is a serious condition that affects people with type 1 diabetes, and occasionally those with type 2 diabetes. In some cases, DKA may be the first sign that someone has diabetes. Some people have ketosis-prone type 2 diabetes. DKA can develop very quickly over several hours.

How is DKA diagnosed?

There are three blood tests used in the diagnosis of DKA.

1 Elevated blood glucose levels (>11 mmol/l): if there is not enough insulin in the body to allow glucose to enter the cells, blood glucose levels will rise (hyperglycaemia). As the body breaks down fat for energy, blood glucose levels will continue to rise.
2 Elevated ketone levels (blood ketones above 3 mmol/l or urine ketones above 2+ on a dipstick): when the body breaks down fat for energy, ketones enter the bloodstream.
3 Blood acidity (pH <7.3 on blood gas analysis; normal pH is 7.35–7.45): excess ketones in the blood cause it to become acidic

Diabetes Care at a Glance, First Edition. Edited by Anne Phillips.
© 2023 John Wiley & Sons Ltd. Published 2023 by John Wiley & Sons Ltd.

(acidosis) and this can change the normal function of organs throughout the body.

Signs and symptoms of DKA
- High blood glucose levels.
- Rapid breathing.
- Being very thirsty.
- Needing to pass urine more often.
- Feeling tired and sleepy.
- Confusion.
- Stomach pain.
- Feeling or being sick.
- Sweet or fruity-smelling breath (like nail polish remover or pear drop sweets).
- Passing out.

What are the triggers that can lead to DKA?
DKA can be triggered by an illness or infection that can cause the body to produce higher levels of certain hormones, such as adrenaline or cortisol. Unfortunately, these hormones act in opposition to the effect of insulin and sometimes trigger an episode of DKA. Examples include chest and urinary tract infections. Sometimes a stressful event such as a heart attack or stroke can be a trigger.

Another issue can be a problem with insulin therapy. Missed insulin doses, not taking enough insulin or a faulty insulin pump can leave a person with insufficient insulin in the body, triggering DKA.

How is DKA treated?
Treatment usually involves the following.

- **Fluid replacement**: most likely intravenous (IV) fluids to replace those lost through excessive urination; also help dilute the excess glucose in the blood.
- **Electrolyte replacement**: electrolytes are salts/minerals (e.g. sodium, potassium, chloride) in the blood that carry an electrical charge. The absence of insulin can lower the level of several electrolytes in the blood. These are initially given intravenously to help keep heart, muscle and nerve cells functioning normally.
- **Insulin therapy**: insulin reverses the processes that cause DKA, and this will initially be given intravenously as well. When blood glucose levels fall to around 11.1 mmol/l and the blood is no longer acidic, the person may be able to stop IV insulin therapy and resume their normal subcutaneous insulin injections.

The underlying cause of the DKA also needs to be managed, for example treating an infection or educating the person about sick day management.

How to avoid DKA
Diabetes can be a stressful condition to live with, but the following are some steps that can reduce the chances of developing DKA.

- Taking diabetes medications or insulin as prescribed and adjusting insulin dosages as needed with the support of diabetes healthcare professionals.
- Medication doses often need adjusting in relation to factors such as blood glucose levels, food, activity and illness.
- People using insulin pumps need to ensure that they have a back-up supply of insulin pens in case the pump stops working.
- Following sick-day management advice is also important. Blood glucose levels should be monitored frequently, and more often during illness or stress. Careful monitoring is the only way to ensure that glucose levels remain within target range.
- Checking ketone levels when hyperglycaemic and during illness or stress. If ketone levels are not reducing with sick-day management, individuals should contact their primary or secondary healthcare professional or seek emergency care.

Hyperosmolar hyperglycaemic state
Hyperosmolar hyperglycaemic state (HHS) is a serious condition that occurs in people with type 2 diabetes who experience very high blood glucose levels (often over 30 mmol/l). It can develop over a course of weeks through a combination of illness (e.g. infection) and dehydration (JBDS-IP 2022). There are some similarities to DKA, but the main symptoms include urination, thirst, nausea, dry skin, disorientation and, in later stages, drowsiness and a gradual loss of consciousness.

Figure 24.1 shows the main features of DKA and HHS.

References
JBDS-IP (2021). The Management of Diabetic Ketoacidosis in Adults. Joint British Diabetes Societies for Inpatient Care, London. Available at https://abcd.care/sites/abcd.care/files/site_uploads/JBDS_Guidelines_Current/JBDS_02%20_DKA_Guideline_amended_v2_June_2021.pdf.
JBDS-IP (2022). The Management of Hyperosmolar Hyperglycaemic State (HHS) in Adults. Joint British Diabetes Societies for Inpatient Care, London. Available at https://abcd.care/resource/jbds-06-management-hyperosmolar-hyperglycaemic-state-hhs-adults-diabetes.

25 Diabetes and steroids

Figure 25.1 Different steroids, doses and duration of action.

Steroid	Potency (equivalent doses)	Duration of action (half-life, in hours)
Hydrocortisone	20 mg	8
Prednisolone	5 mg	16–36
Methylprednisolone	4 mg	18–40
Dexamethasone	0.75 mg	36–54
Betamethasone	0.75 mg	26–54

Figure 25.2 The effect of corticosteroids on blood glucose.

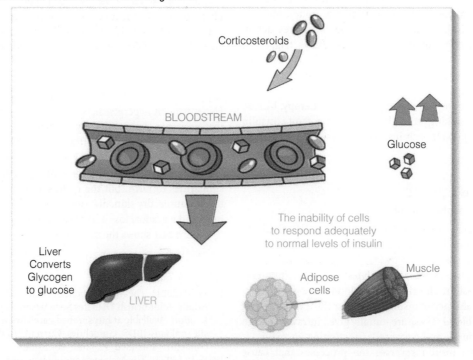

Figure 25.3 Risk factors for steroid-induced diabetes.

Risk factors of steroid-induced diabetes

There are some factors that may mean you are more likely to develop diabetes if you are taking steroids. These include if you:

- are over 40 and white, or over 25 and African-Caribbean, Black African or South Asian
- have a close family member with type 2 diabetes
- are of African-Caribbean, Black African or South Asian descent
- have had high blood pressure
- are living with obesity.

Diabetes Care at a Glance, First Edition. Edited by Anne Phillips.
© 2023 John Wiley & Sons Ltd. Published 2023 by John Wiley & Sons Ltd.

What are steroids?

Steroids are also known as corticosteroids. They are artificial versions of hormones that are naturally produced by the body. They reduce inflammation and can help to treat a wide range of conditions, including:

- severe asthma
- cystic fibrosis
- arthritis
- inflammatory bowel disease
- some types of cancers.
    (Note that these are different from anabolic steroids.)

Different steroids

There are different types of steroids, which can be prescribed in many forms. High doses of steroids are often taken orally or as an injection and are more likely to affect blood glucose levels. Some people with diabetes are also being treated for various inflammatory conditions with steroids such as dexamethasone, hydrocortisone, prednisolone and intravenous methylprednisolone. More recently, dexamethasone has been used in the management of COVID-19 (Diabetes UK 2020; National Institute for Health and Care Excellence 2021). Figure 25.1 provides a list of widely used corticosteroids and their equivalent doses and duration of action.

Steroid-induced hyperglycaemia or steroid-induced diabetes

A rise in glucose related to steroid therapy occurring in people without a known diagnosis of diabetes is termed steroid-induced diabetes. The use of steroid treatment in people with pre-existing diabetes will undoubtedly result in worsening glucose control; this may be termed steroid-induced hyperglycaemia.

How do steroids cause steroid-induced diabetes?

Steroids increase blood glucose levels in two ways.
- They reduce the body's sensitivity to insulin by reducing the ability of muscle and fat (adipose) cells to absorb glucose from the blood (known as insulin resistance).
- They cause the liver to release stored glucose, even when the body does not need additional glucose.
    Figure 25.2 shows how steroids impact blood glucose levels.

Is steroid-induced diabetes permanent?

Many people will find that their blood glucose levels return to a healthy range when they stop taking steroids. For others, however, steroid-induced diabetes can continue even after stopping their treatment. This is more likely if they are at higher risk of developing type 2 diabetes. The risk factors for type 2 diabetes are shown in Figure 25.3.

Signs and symptoms of steroid-induced diabetes

Patients taking steroids, but who are not monitoring their blood glucose, will need to be aware of the symptoms of hyperglycaemia. These are the same as the symptoms of undiagnosed diabetes (discussed in Chapter 3), which include:

- excessive thirst
- excessive urination
- feeling very tired
- possibly losing weight unintentionally.

People who are already monitoring their blood glucose may need to increase the frequency or adjust their medication with the support of their diabetes primary or secondary care teams. If no action is taken, the individual may develop acute and long-term complications associated with hyperglycaemia.

How is it diagnosed?

The diagnostic criteria for steroid-induced hyperglycaemia do not differ from those for other types of diabetes and include a confirmed fasting venous blood glucose of 7 mmol/l or above, a random venous glucose level of 11.1 mmol/l or above, or two or more capillary blood glucose levels above 12 mmol/l. When people are in hospital, there will be specific guidelines on how to identify and manage steroid-induced diabetes (Joint British Diabetes Societies for In-patient Care 2021).

Treatment of steroid-induced hyperglycaemia

Treatment needs to be individualized, for example length of the course of steroids and the steroid dose. Sulfonylureas (SUs) such as gliclazide and glipizide are often used to tackle mild steroid-induced hyperglycaemia (Chapter 14 discusses different oral diabetes therapies). SUs stimulate the pancreas to release insulin and are best suited to manage the peaks in glucose caused by steroids. People who start taking SUs need to be provided with a blood glucose monitor and receive education in how to use it. They need to monitor their blood glucose levels regularly and be in contact with diabetes primary or secondary care teams for advice on whether they need to adjust their dose. Monitoring also helps them to detect hypoglycaemia (low blood glucose levels). There is an increased risk of hypoglycaemia with SUs, especially when steroid doses are tapered or if meals are skipped. Part of their education therefore needs to include how to manage hypoglycaemia.

In those with significant hyperglycaemia, some people may need to start insulin. Insulin has the benefit of having an immediate onset of action and doses can be increased regularly to an effective dose. These people will require education regarding insulin injection technique, blood glucose monitoring, adjustment of insulin, and recognition and management of hypoglycaemia. The insulin type will depend on the steroid and frequency of dose. For example, morning administration of an intermediate-acting insulin such as Humulin I may closely fit the glucose peaks during late afternoon to evening induced by a single dose of oral steroid in the morning. A basal analogue insulin such as Lantus may be appropriate if hyperglycaemia is present throughout the day and into the evening.

References

Diabetes UK (2020). Diabetes when you're unwell. www.diabetes. org.uk/guide-to-diabetes/life-with-diabetes/illness (accessed 18 February 2021).

National Institute for Health and Care Excellence (2021). Therapeutics for COVID-19: corticosteroids. In: COVID-19 Rapid Guideline: Managing COVID-19. NICE Guideline NG191. www.nice.org.uk/guidance/ng191 (accessed 15 June 2022).

Joint British Diabetes Societies for In-patient Care (JBDS-IP) (2021). Management of Hyperglycaemia and Steroid (Glucocorticoid) Therapy. https://abcd.care/sites/abcd.care/files/site_uploads/ JBDS_Guidelines_Current/JBDS_08_Steroids_DM_Guideline_ FINAL_28052021.pdf (accessed 27 April 2022).

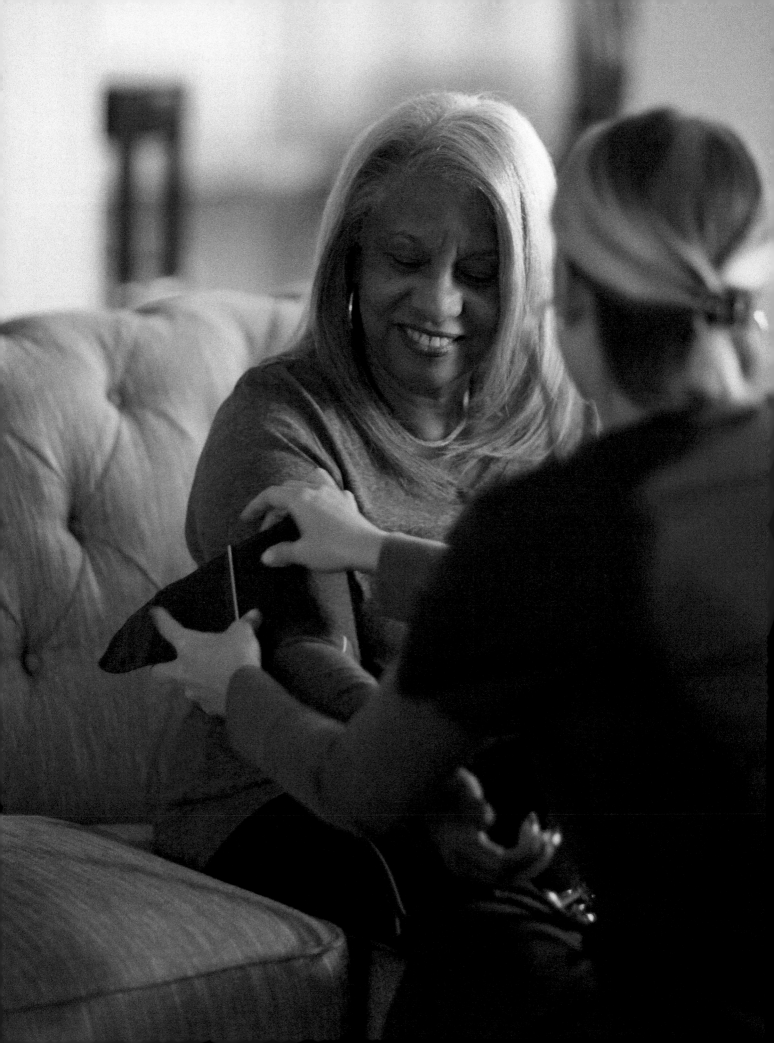

Life stages

Part 5

Chapters

26 Transition

Figure 26.1 Changing from children to young people.

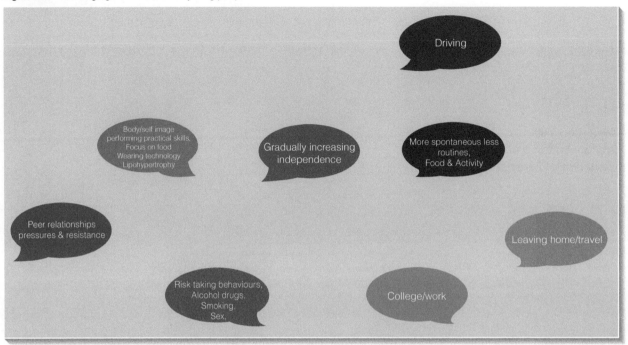

Figure 26.2 The ladder of participation in transitional care.

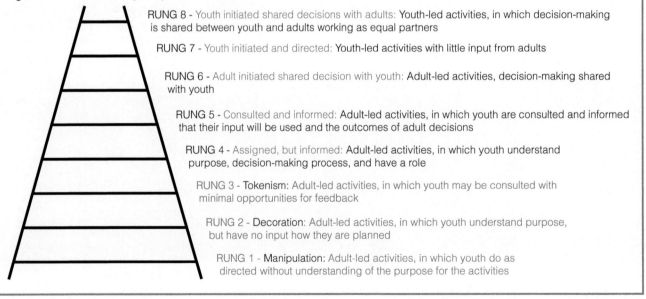

RUNG 8 - Youth initiated shared decisions with adults: Youth-led activities, in which decision-making is shared between youth and adults working as equal partners

RUNG 7 - Youth initiated and directed: Youth-led activities with little input from adults

RUNG 6 - Adult initiated shared decision with youth: Adult-led activities, decision-making shared with youth

RUNG 5 - Consulted and informed: Adult-led activities, in which youth are consulted and informed that their input will be used and the outcomes of adult decisions

RUNG 4 - Assigned, but informed: Adult-led activities, in which youth understand purpose, decision-making process, and have a role

RUNG 3 - Tokenism: Adult-led activities, in which youth may be consulted with minimal opportunities for feedback

RUNG 2 - Decoration: Adult-led activities, in which youth understand purpose, but have no input how they are planned

RUNG 1 - Manipulation: Adult-led activities, in which youth do as directed without understanding of the purpose for the activities

Diabetes Care at a Glance, First Edition. Edited by Anne Phillips.
© 2023 John Wiley & Sons Ltd. Published 2023 by John Wiley & Sons Ltd.

Transition has been defined as the 'purposeful, planned movement of adolescent and young adults with long term medical conditions from child-centred to adult orientated health care systems' (Blum et al. 1993). Creating the right culture for securing full participation of young people in this process is fundamental.

Given the increasing prevalence of all types of diabetes, the higher mortality among 10–19 year olds, that 10% of young people will develop microvascular complications, that almost half will need psychological support, that significant numbers are lost to follow-up once they leave paediatric care and concerns that suboptimal HbA1c may lead to increased risk of long-term complications and impact on quality of life, effective transition must be prioritized. As behaviours set down in adolescence are generally carried through to adulthood, healthcare professionals have a narrow window of opportunity to get transitional care right for young people. Calls to extend services up to 25 years of age have also been made and are gathering momentum.

During puberty and up to the mid-twenties the body and brain continue to develop and mature. Puberty and growth are associated with increased insulin requirements and insulin resistance with a marked dawn phenomenon, which can compound the developmental challenges experienced. In addition to the physical changes, the brain continues to develop during adolescence, with research suggesting that the prefrontal cortex, important in planning, prioritizing and complex decision-making, is the last to mature (Blakemore 2012). Consequently, spontaneity and risk-taking behaviours such as unplanned sleepovers, sex, alcohol and driving can impact diabetes and increase the risk of hypoglycaemia and hyperglycaemia (Figure 26.1). Furthermore, time spent with glucose levels above range, perhaps due to omitting insulin and then reacting by giving large boluses separate to food intake or several smaller boluses in quick succession, which can cause insulin to accumulate, exacerbate the risk of hypoglycaemia.

With such challenges, as well as the relentless focus on food, it is not surprising that type 1 diabetes and eating disorders (T1DE) often emerges in adolescence. Asking young people about T1DE and assessing risk with a validated tool is important in ensuring early referral when required to mental health teams and in facilitating integrated working to provide tailored support and intervention.

Transition coordinator roles and continuity in care can support and strengthen the therapeutic relationship. Meeting the young-adult team before transfer followed by two to three appointments in timely succession may help to build rapport. Offering young people time by themselves from the age of 12 to help prepare for self-care is also recommended. If young people do not attend secondary care services, effective communication and integrated care pathways with primary care will be needed.

Interactive structured education programmes include topics specific to this developmental stage and rites of passage that encourage informal, fun conversations with peers and facilitators around sensitive topics. NHS-approved platforms such as https://www.digibete.org/ and My diabetes My way (https://diabetesmyway.nhs.uk/) support consistent and accessible person-centred digital education. The Ready Steady Go Transition Programme (2022) helps to gradually empower young people by equipping them with the knowledge and skills to confidently manage their own health in order to smoothly move from paediatric to adult services. Young people should be actively involved throughout the transition process as an equal partner in decision-making. Full participation has the potential to reduce health inequalities and social exclusion, leading to more effective services as well as empowering young people.

Models and frameworks for participation enable us to recognize where healthcare professionals, the team and the service are on the ladder of participation (Figure 26.2) and work towards increasing this further, with the top rung achieving youth-initiated shared decisions. Actively seeking feedback from young people is recognized as key in creating a continuous cycle of improvement within the transition service.

Listening to the individual's story is important in understanding the person's experience of living with diabetes and building a rapport to aid recognition of any specific challenges, needs and concerns while equally acknowledging resilience and burnout. Some young people will be ready and confident for this next phase of their journey and will embrace the increased responsibilities and freedoms of moving away from the family home to study or work. In contrast, for others this change may heighten anxiety. For those with additional physical or learning needs, levels of confidence and readiness may also vary. Adapting or differentiating certain aspects of the pathway to facilitate engagement and participation may be needed.

The level of participation for young people experiencing health inequalities due to social deprivation, culture, race and ethnicity must also be considered. Digital educational resources are increasingly available in different languages, and transcription features on virtual learning platforms can also help widen access and engagement in addition to interpreting services.

Renegotiating and maintaining parental involvement through adolescence has been associated with improved health outcomes during this vulnerable stage, so reviewing this at each contact is important in reducing the risk of diabetes burnout and deterioration in glycaemic control. Some young people may prefer to bring along a supportive friend, which should also be encouraged.

Sustaining and continuing to build on the young person's self-care and autonomy so they can reach their full potential and lead a fulfilling and complication-free life is fundamental.

References

Blakemore, S.-J. (2012). Development of the social brain in adolescence. *J. R. Soc. Med.* 105 (3): 111–116. https://doi.org/10.1258/jrsm.2011.110221.

Blum, R.W., Garell, D., Hodgman, C.H. et al. (1993). Transition from child-centered to adult health-care systems for adolescents with chronic conditions. A position paper of the Society for Adolescent Medicine. *J. Adolesc. Health* 14 (7): 570–576. https://doi.org/10.1016/1054-139x(93)90143-d.

Ready Steady Go Transition Programme (2022). https://www.uhs.nhs.uk/for-visitors/southampton-childrens-hospital/childrens-services/ready-steady-go-transition-programme.

27 Preconception care and diabetes

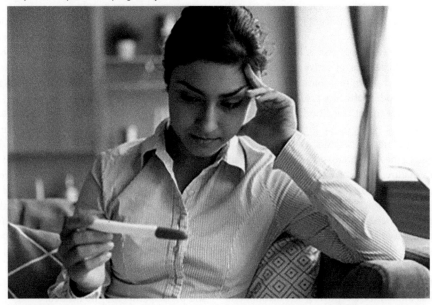

Figure 27.1 Diabetes in preconception and pregnancy. *Source:* fizkes/Adobe Stock.

Before insulin was used to treat people with diabetes, women were described as giving birth over a grave. It was rare for women with type 1 diabetes to become pregnant and without insulin sadly the woman and the baby rarely survived. Since 1922 when insulin treatment for diabetes began, the outcomes for both mother and baby have improved dramatically. Nevertheless, women with type 1 or type 2 diabetes are still at higher risk of a stillbirth, neonatal death or baby born with congenital anomalies (Figure 27.1).

These risks can be reduced by good preconception care. Preconception care is often done in a dedicated clinic that can review diabetes and obstetric history, screen for complications and reduce risks related to pregnancy by prescribing safe medication and optimizing glycaemic control. High blood glucose levels can cause problems with the development of organs in the fetus, and these organs start to develop in the first weeks of pregnancy, often before a woman may know that she is pregnant. These congenital anomalies are most commonly cardiac, skeletal or neural tube defects. Although unable to eliminate all risk of miscarriage, congenital malformation, stillbirth and neonatal death, risk will be reduced if a woman planning pregnancy has good glucose control before conception and throughout the pregnancy. It is therefore crucial that women of childbearing age are made aware of the importance of preconception care and the importance of reliable contraception if not planning pregnancy.

Guidance from the National Institute for Health and Care Excellence (2015) is that women with diabetes should aim for an HbA1c of less than 48 mmol/mol (6.5%) but any reduction in HbA1c will reduce risk. However, women with an HbA1c of 86 mmol/mol (10.0%) should be counselled not to become pregnant because of the increased risk due to the high glycaemia. If women are not already testing for glucose control, they should be encouraged to do so. The NICE (2015) guidance for pregnancy is for fasting blood glucose levels to be less than 5.3 mmol/l and at one hour post meals to be less than 7.8 mmol/l. Women may find real-time continuous glucose monitoring (rtCGM) or intermittently scanned continuous glucose monitoring (isCGM) helpful not only in reducing the burden of fingerprick testing but also in assessing the fluctuating glucose levels over 24 hours and reducing the risk of hypoglycaemia.

For women with type 2 diabetes, all non-insulin medication apart from metformin should be stopped prior to conception due to concerns or lack of evidence about other diabetes medication being used in pregnancy. For many women with type 2 diabetes this will necessitate them taking insulin prior to conception to meet their glycaemic target levels; for most such women this will involve a basal-bolus regimen comprising rapid-acting insulin at mealtimes and an intermediate or long-acting insulin as background insulin. This allows greater flexibility and the ability to manipulate the insulin to target specific times where glucose levels may be difficult to control.

Women with type 1 diabetes should normally have received structured education regarding carbohydrate counting and management of diabetes, for example Dose Adjustment For Normal Eating (DAFNE). These women should be using multiple injections of rapid-acting insulin to match carbohydrate intake/glucose level and background insulin once or twice a day; alternatively, many women benefit from an insulin pump and ideally this should be done prior to pregnancy so that they can get used to the pump and stabilized on it prior to conception.

Folic acid can reduce the risk of neural tube defects and should be taken by all women planning pregnancy. As women with diabetes are at increased risk, they should be advised to take a higher dose of folic acid (5 mg once daily). This dose is only available on prescription in the UK. Women should be advised to take it for at least three months prior to conceiving and then for the first 12 weeks of pregnancy.

When a woman is contemplating pregnancy the medications that she is on should be reviewed. Oral diabetes medications or non-insulin injectables should be stopped and converted to insulin. Statins should be stopped, and other medications commonly used in people with diabetes, such as angiotensin-converting enzyme (ACE) inhibitors and angiotensin II receptor antagonists, should be stopped and changed to medications that are safe to use in pregnancy.

Being overweight or obese can impact and reduce a woman's fertility. It can also affect diabetes control and make it more difficult to reach glycaemic targets and can also increase risk of complications in pregnancy, including an increased risk of late fetal and neonatal death. Therefore, it is important to discuss healthy eating and physical activity prior to conception in order to maximize chance of conception and reduce weight.

Hypoglycaemia is a concern for both women with diabetes and health professionals. Trying to reach tight glycaemic targets can be difficult and may increase the risk of hypoglycaemia. In addition, women in early pregnancy often find that their blood glucose levels drop, precipitating hypoglycaemia. It is therefore important prior to a woman becoming pregnant to discuss the causes, symptoms, treatment and management of hypoglycaemia with them, ensuring that their own practice is current and safe. Teaching how to administer glucagon to a partner or family member can also be beneficial in case hypoglycaemia is severe. There needs to be discussion and agreement on safe individualized glycaemic targets to optimize glycaemic control but without frequent or severe hypoglycaemia. rtCGM or isCGM may also be useful, especially in women who may have reduced hypoglycaemia awareness.

Preconception care for women with diabetes has been proven to reduce risk associated with diabetes and pregnancy. All women with diabetes need to be made aware of this, at every opportunity, to raise awareness and improve lives.

Reference

National Institute for Health and Care Excellence (2015). Diabetes in Pregnancy: Management from Preconception to the Postnatal Period. NICE Guidance NG3. Last updated December 2020. Available at https://www.nice.org.uk/guidance/ng3

28 Gestational diabetes

Figure 28.1 Gestational diabetes. *Source:* Наталия Кузина / Adobe Stock.

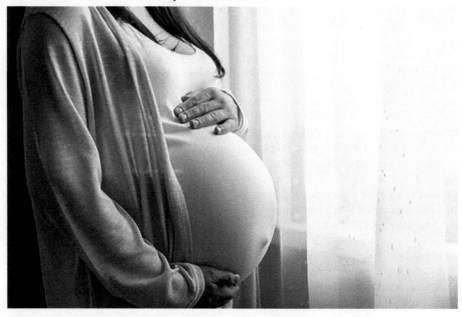

Figure 28.2 NICE NG3 Guidance 2015.

NICE National Institute for
Health and Care Excellence

NICE

guideline

Diabetes in pregnancy: management from preconception to the postnatal period

NICE guideline
Published: 25 February 2015
nice.org.uk/guidance/ng3

Gestational diabetes (GDM) is diabetes that develops during pregnancy and which usually resolves after giving birth. It can happen at any stage of pregnancy but is more likely to occur in the second or third trimester of pregnancy (Figure 28.1). GDM is the commonest type of diabetes in pregnancy, affecting 5–25% of all pregnant women depending on the diagnostic criteria used.

The higher-than-normal blood glucose levels can have implications for the mother and the baby. With GDM there is a small increase in the risk of serious birth complications, including macrosomia (large baby), problems with birth and delivery including birth trauma, neonatal hypoglycaemia and perinatal death. Children of mothers with GDM have higher rates of overweight and obesity by 11 years of age, which can lead to the child developing type 2 diabetes later in life (National Institute for Health and Care Excellence (2015) (Figure 28.2). Careful monitoring and treatment can reduce these risks.

GDM may not cause any symptoms, so it is important that women who are at risk of GDM are screened. Women who are at risk include those with:

- body mass index (BMI) above 30 kg/m²
- a previous macrosomic baby weighing 4.5 kg or above
- previous gestational diabetes
- a first-degree relative with diabetes
- an ethnicity with a high prevalence of diabetes.

Women should also be considered at risk if they have had glycosuria 2+ or above on one occasion or 1+ or above on two or more occasions.

Screening and diagnosis of GDM normally involves a 75-g two-hour oral glucose tolerance test (OGTT) at around 24–28 weeks of pregnancy in which the woman is fasted and her fasting blood glucose level and the blood glucose response to a 75-g glucose drink are measured. According to NICE (2015), gestational diabetes is diagnosed if there is:

- a fasting plasma glucose level of 5.6 mmol/l or above, or
- a two-hour plasma glucose level of 7.8 mmol/l or above.

Women who have had previous GDM may be offered an early OGTT as soon as possible after booking and again at 24–28 weeks if the first OGTT results are within range. Alternatively, women who have a previous history of GDM can be offered early self-monitoring of blood glucose levels. This is because these women are likely to develop GDM again in subsequent pregnancies or may have developed type 2 diabetes in the interim.

All women with GDM should be taught how to monitor their own blood glucose levels. The target blood glucose levels for GDM are the same as those for women with pre-gestational diabetes:

- fasting blood glucose levels less than 5.3 mmol/l
- one-hour post meal levels less than 7.8 mmol/l.

Initially, women are asked to check their blood glucose levels at least four times daily: before breakfast and then one hour after meals.

A woman who is diagnosed with GDM should be given an explanation of the implications for her pregnancy and beyond and be allowed to discuss this with a healthcare professional. It can be an extremely anxious time so the woman should be reassured that good glucose control by self-monitoring throughout pregnancy can help to reduce risks.

Diet is extremely important in helping to manage glucose control in pregnancy. Women with GDM need advice and support on choosing the right sorts of food. Carbohydrate is important in supplying sufficient energy and nutrition to support a healthy pregnancy; however, excessive carbohydrate can make it impossible to maintain glucose levels within a normal range. Therefore, eating smaller amounts of carbohydrates and choosing carbohydrates that are more likely to create a slower and lower rise in glucose levels after eating can make a significant difference. For example, changing from white flour-based foods to whole-wheat products can help. In order to help fasting blood glucose levels it is also advisable to avoid carbohydrate late in the evening/night. Eating more vegetables and protein foods such as eggs, meat, fish, cheese and pulses can help to prevent the rise in post-meal glucose levels and also help with satiety after a meal.

Activity is also important: for example, going for a walk following a meal, can reduce post-meal glucose by as much as 2 mmol/l.

Medication is normally started if after one week of dietary changes three or more blood glucose levels are raised. Only metformin or insulin is used to treat diabetes in pregnancy. Metformin, if not contraindicated, is started first, normally 500 mg twice daily and titrated to 1 g twice daily if required and tolerated. Modified-release metformin may help if a woman experiences gastrointestinal side effects. If metformin is not tolerated or if after metformin 1 g twice daily blood glucose levels remain raised, then insulin should be added. Normally insulin is started according to the level blood glucose is above target.

A frequent occurrence in GDM is a raised blood glucose level following breakfast, so rapid-acting insulin given with breakfast may help to target this. However, if other readings are above target, then often a basal-bolus insulin regimen is required whereby rapid insulin is given with food to target the post-meal blood glucose levels and isophone/long-acting insulin is given at night to target raised fasting blood glucose levels. The woman will need to be educated in all aspects of insulin use, including how to administer the insulin, hypoglycaemia and driving advice. Close contact is required, either virtually or face to face, to ensure insulin is adjusted according to blood glucose levels as during the second and third trimester insulin requirements are likely to increase.

Once the placenta is delivered, blood glucose levels are likely to return to normal. However, type 2 diabetes can be acquired during pregnancy, so it is important that women are checked postnatally to ensure that the diabetes has disappeared, normally with a three-month HbA1c test.

Women who have had GDM are approximately 10 times more likely to develop type 2 diabetes. Maintaining a healthy weight and being active can help to reduce this risk or prolong the time it takes to develop diabetes. They should also be advised to undergo an annual HbA1c test to screen for diabetes and ensure that, if discovered, it is managed promptly to reduce the risk of long-term complications.

Reference

National Institute for Health and Care Excellence (2015). Diabetes in Pregnancy: Management from Preconception to the Postnatal Period. NICE Guidance NG3. Last updated December 2020. Available at https://www.nice.org.uk/guidance/ng3

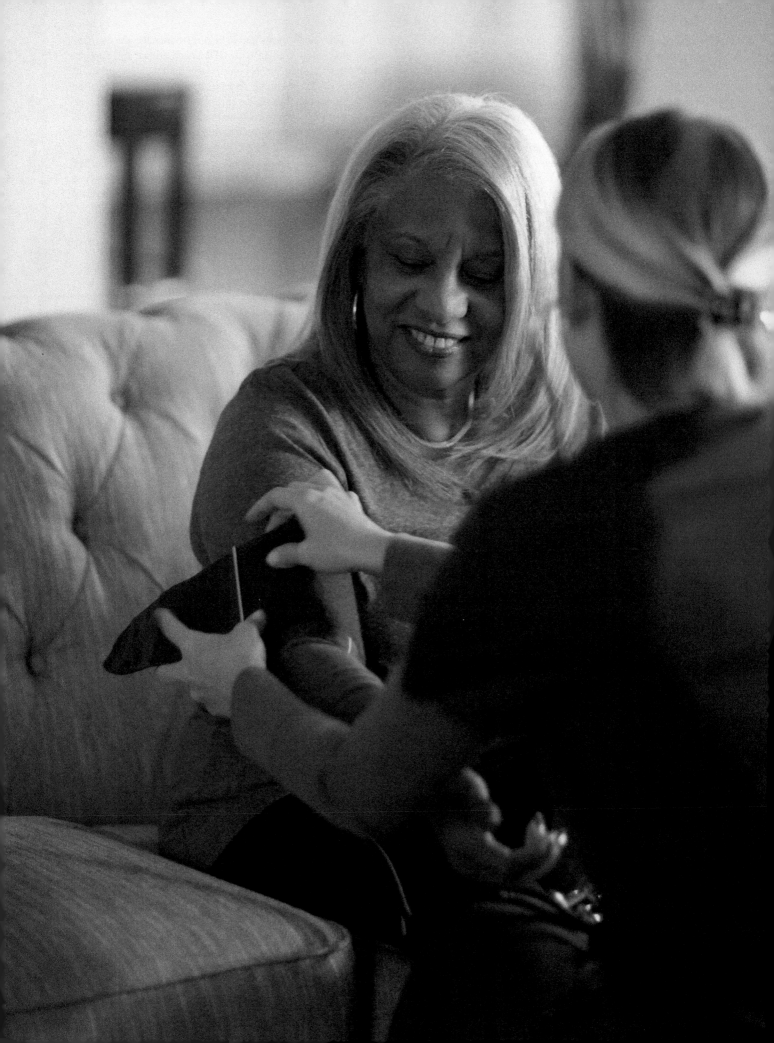

Complications

Part 6

29 Annual reviews in diabetes care

Figure 29.1 Pathology tests assessed at annual reviews.

- HbA1c to assess glucose control over the last 6–8 weeks
- Full blood count to ensure HbA1c result is not affected by anaemia
- Serum B12 as diabetes can affect this
- Urea and electrolytes to assess renal function
- Liver function tests to screen and monitor liver disease
- Thyroid function test to screen for thyroid disorders
- Serum lipid levels to measure cholesterol
- Serum total protein level to assess renal functioning
- Urine albumin/creatinine ratio to assess renal function
- Urine protein levels to assess renal function
- eGFR to screen for evidence of kidney dysfunction

Figure 29.2 Diabetes UK 9 key care processes.

The 9 key processes of care measurements are:

1. Weight and BMI
2. Blood pressure
3. HbA1c
4. Retinopathy screening
5. Foot risk stratification
6. Urinary albumin test
7. Serum creatinine
8. Smoking status
9. Cholesterol level

Figure 29.3 LET'S TALK NOW pre-diabetes review helpful patient guide.

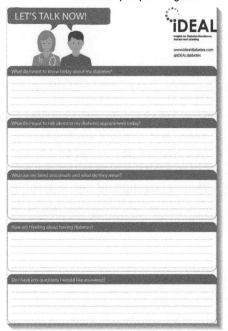

Figure 29.4 Annual and interim diabetes review record sheet to share with the individual.

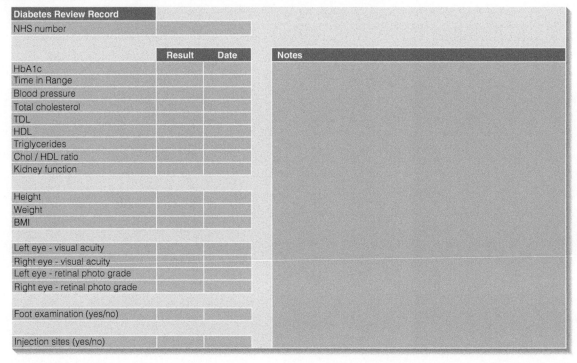

Diabetes Review Record			
NHS number			
	Result	**Date**	**Notes**
HbA1c			
Time in Range			
Blood pressure			
Total cholesterol			
TDL			
HDL			
Triglycerides			
Chol / HDL ratio			
Kidney function			
Height			
Weight			
BMI			
Left eye - visual acuity			
Right eye - visual acuity			
Left eye - retinal photo grade			
Right eye - retinal photo grade			
Foot examination (yes/no)			
Injection sites (yes/no)			

Diabetes Care at a Glance, First Edition. Edited by Anne Phillips.
© 2023 John Wiley & Sons Ltd. Published 2023 by John Wiley & Sons Ltd.

All people with diabetes should undergo a diabetes care review at least annually. The ideal review for those aged over 19 years is an annual review and a six-monthly interim review. Children and young people should be reviewed every three months and pregnant women more frequently due to pregnancy.

The diabetes review is part of the process whereby each individual's health, including their blood pressure, cholesterol levels and medications, is reassessed. The blood and urine tests required and the rationale for their inclusion in the annual review are detailed in Figure 29.1. The annual review is based on Diabetes UK 9 Health Key Essentials (Figure 29.2) and these are collected annually by the NHS to measure the quality of diabetes care provided and the impact across every region in the UK in the National Diabetes Audit (2022).

Diabetes is a long-term and progressive condition that can potentially have damaging effects on an individual's health. However, evidence shows that many of the complications associated with diabetes can be prevented or delayed through a combination of foot and eye screening, attending appointments with a healthcare professional, learning to self-managing diabetes, and the appropriate use of medicines and technology (i.e. diabetes education, blood glucose meters, home testing of blood pressure and understanding the results). Therefore, annual assessment of these processes of care is important.

It is recommended that people are helped to prepare for their annual review and to use a prompt to enable individuals to ask the questions we would like them to be able to ask in their review. Encouraging people to be a partner in their diabetes review is fundamental as it is their review and not the health professional's. Preparing a list of questions or topics to discuss is always useful so it is recommended to introduce this to everyone with diabetes at diagnosis and before each annual and interim review. An ideal approach is to use the LET'S TALK NOW approach (Figure 29.3).

At the annual review the activities shown in Figure 29.4 will be undertaken. People can see their annual review as like a vehicle MOT. The annual review is a health review but can also be seen as an opportunity to screen for potential complications so needs to be undertaken with rigour but also in a person-centred way. Because of the complexity of both type 1 and type 2 diabetes, it can be helpful to undertake medication review and optimization at the annual and interim reviews.

The annual and interim reviews are opportunities to offer educational updates to make every contact count (NHS Health Education England 2022). The annual review also offers opportunities for utilizing information prescriptions for each individual depending on their goals and health needs (see Chapter 10). Care planning is part of a person-centred approach and can help people be more actively involved in their care decisions and goal setting (see Chapter 12). Some core principles of this approach require the clinician to 'set aside' their professional expert persona and to work as a partner with each individual in their diabetes care decisions. Such an approach can encourage people to share and discuss information and issues that may be bothering them (Figure 29.3).

It can be helpful to present information in different ways for individuals, such as using cardiovascular risk calculators or patient decision aids. Sensitive questioning relating to psychological health and sexual health, mood and relationships can provide the opportunity for patients to be listened to and appropriate treatments to be facilitated. It is important to use the right language approaches (see Chapter 4) and to promote inclusivity in decision-making to enable 'No decision about me, without me' (Department of Health 2012).

The diabetes review is an opportunity to monitor each individual's diabetes care and to share and discuss information and results in a person-centred way. The aim of the results is to support people in the prevention of acute and longer-term complications. Information relating to risk is part of the review and can be communicated in an individualized way and in a way that enables people with diabetes to make decisions and choices about their diabetes care.

References

Department of Health (2012). Liberating the NHS: No Decision About Me Without Me. Available at https://assets.publishing.service.gov.uk/government/uploads/system/uploads/attachment_data/file/216980/Liberating-the-NHS-No-decision-about-me-without-me-Government-response.pdf.

NHS Health Education England (2022). Making every contact count. www.makingeverycontactcount.co.uk.

NHS Digital National Diabetes Audit (2022). https://digital.nhs.uk/data-and-information/publications/statistical/national-diabetes-audit.

30 Neurovascular foot assessment

Figure 30.1 Palpation of pedal pulses: (a) dorsalis pedis artery; (b) posterior tibial artery.

(a)

(b)

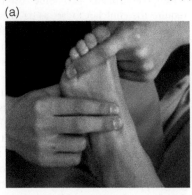

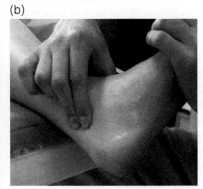

Figure 30.2 Using Doppler ultrasound in vascular assessment (shown here in an ankle/brachial pressure index assessment). *Source:* Courtesy of Edmonds and Foster (2005).

Figure 30.3 Using a 10-g monofilament for neurological assessment.

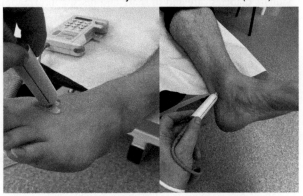

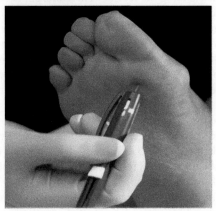

Figure 30.4 Risk stratification tool. *Source:* The University of Edinburgh, www.diabetesframe.org/nhs-scotland/03-the-purpose-of-foot-screening-nhs-scotland/risk-stratification-low-risk/.

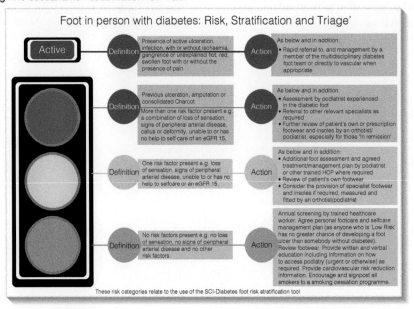

This chapter shows how a neurovascular assessment is performed in order to determine the nerve and blood supply to the foot in people with diabetes. Early monitoring of the nerve supply and circulation in a person with diabetes is essential for the assessment and prevention of foot problems, including ulceration and amputation.

The procedure for performing a simple annual foot check is detailed in Figures 30.1 and 30.3, all people with diabetes should have this carried out by a healthcare practitioner to avoid the risk of foot problems developing.

Vascular assessment

As the feet are the body part furthest from the heart, blood has the longest distance to travel and blockages may occur that reduce the blood flow, leading to pain in the feet/legs when walking (intermittent claudication) or at rest (rest pain) with associated tissue changes (ulceration/necrosis/gangrene). Blood flow to the feet can be assessed by palpating the foot pulses (Figure 30.1) or listening to the blood flow with a Doppler ultrasound device (Figure 30.2). If the pulses are not palpable, then consider referral to a vascular specialist for further investigation, especially if the patient has any symptoms or has any wounds on their feet.

Peripheral neuropathy

There are three main types of neuropathy affecting people with diabetes: sensory, motor and autonomic. Most people develop loss of peripheral pain sensation (sensory neuropathy), and are often completely unaware of its presence. It is vitally important therefore to regularly assess for loss of sensation as this may result in the inability to feel pain, or hot and cold, with the result that injury often occurs. This loss of the protective pain sensation can be assessed in the clinic or home environment using a 10-g monofilament (Figure 30.3) or the Ipswich Touch Test (Rayman et al. 2011). The assessment should take place in a quiet environment with the patient lying or sitting and with their eyes closed.

The 10-g monofilament should be applied at 90°, perpendicular to the surface of the skin, until it bends. The person's response should be noted. The four testing sites are:

- plantar aspect of the great toe
- plantar aspect of the middle toe
- plantar aspect of the little toe
- plantar aspect of the first metatarsal head.

Sites may vary according to local guidelines.

The Ipswich Touch Test is similar in that the patient is asked to close their eyes while the healthcare practitioner places an index finger one at a time on the tips of the first, third and fifth toes (for two seconds) on each foot. The patient is asked to respond 'yes' when they feel this touch. Sensory neuropathy is determined where there are more than two 'no' responses out of the six locations tested. This test has been found to be as sensitive and specific as the 10-g monofilament for detecting peripheral sensory neuropathy and requires no equipment.

Failure to feel any sensation indicates sensory loss, although some sites may be felt and others not, which is known as 'patchy' neuropathy.

Carrying out a neurovascular assessment enables the rapid detection of foot problems and so facilitates early referral for further intervention and/or treatment if the patient is deemed to be at increased risk of ulceration (Rawles 2014). The person with diabetes should be informed of their results and what it means for them.

The risk stratification tool illustrated in Figure 30.4 enables a patient's risk of ulceration to be assessed based on their neurovascular assessment and builds sequentially, with all patients receiving education and emergency contact details regardless of their risk category as many people with diabetes will have 'lost the gift of pain' (Boulton 2013) as a result of neuropathy, and so will be less likely to know when they have a foot problem or when or indeed where to seek foot health advice and treatment.

References

Boulton, A.J.M. (2013). The pathway to foot ulceration in diabetes. *Med. Clin. North Am.* 97 (5): 775–790. https://doi.org/10.1016/j.mcna.2013.03.007.

Rawles, Z. (2014). Assessing the foot in patients with diabetes. *Nursing Times* 110 (31): 20–22.

Rayman, G., Vas, P.R., Baker, N. et al. (2011). The Ipswich Touch Test. *Diabetes Care* 34 (7): 1517–1518.

Edmonds, M., and Foster, A. (2015). *Managing the Diabetic Foot*, 2nd Ed. UK: Wiley Blackwell.

Further reading

Edmonds, M., Phillips, A., Holmes, P. et al. (2020). To halve the number of major amputations in people living with diabetes, 'ACT NOW'. *Diabetes Prim. Care* 22 (6): 139–143. http://bit.ly/3pLHMDo.

Masson, E. (2017). Neuropathic presentations in diabetes. In: *Principles of Diabetes Care: Evidence Based Practice for Health Professionals* (ed. A. Phillips), chapter 20. Salisbury: Quay Books.

National Institute for Health and Care Excellence (2015). Diabetic Foot Problems: Prevention and Management. NICE Guideline NG19. www.nice.org.uk/guidance/ng19 (accessed 26 May 2021).

Phillips, A. and Mehl, A. (2015). Diabetes mellitus and the increased risk of foot injuries. *J. Wound Care* 24 (5): 4–7.

31 ACT NOW: A foot assessment tool

Figure 31.1 The ACT NOW infographic explained.

ACT NOW

A Accident (Recent, to foot or toe)

C Change (In colour or shape of foot or toes)

T Temperature (Change in foot or toes, hotter or colder)

N New pain (In foot or toes)

O Oozing (From area of skin or nail on foot or toes)

W Wound (New blister or skin break, may be under toenail or corn)

Figure 31.2 The ACT NOW checklist, with additional prompts regarding the six steps as well as areas for date and clinical photographs (with patient consent) that enables the tool to be used as part of patient's referral or ongoing management plan. *Source:* Adapted from https://www.diabetes.org.uk/guide-to-diabetes/.

ACT NOW!

Tool for all NHS Primary and Secondary Care services to promote prompt and rapid referral to the MDFT (Multidisciplinary Foot Care Team) (Edmonds et al, 2020).

Refer the PWD (Person/People With Diabetes) if they present with any of the following to their foot/feet:

ACT NOW!
Checklist

ASSESSMENT OF FOOT	Tick if present	Digital photo taken to include with referral	Date referred	Document referral to Specialist MDFT
A - ACCIDENT? Recent or history of an accident or trauma?				
C - CHANGE? Is there any new swelling, redness or change of shape of the foot?				
T - TEMPERATURE? If there is a change in temperature present? Could this be an infection or possible Charcot?				
N - NEW PAIN? Is there pain present? Is it localised or generalised throughtout the foot?				
O - OOZING? What color is any exudate? Is there an odour?				
W - WOUND? Can you document the size, type and position of the wound in the foot affected?				

Diabetes Care at a Glance, First Edition. Edited by Anne Phillips.
© 2023 John Wiley & Sons Ltd. Published 2023 by John Wiley & Sons Ltd.

Figure 31.3 The ACT NOW infographic.

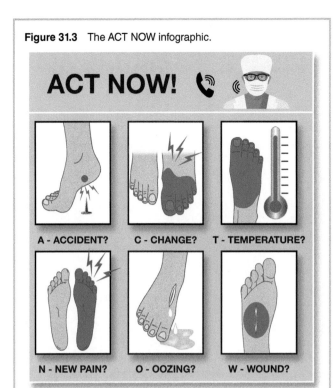

This chapter introduces the ACT NOW toolkit, comprising the checklist and infographic, and provides the information needed to use this simple, practical, six-step resource in order to recognize the warning signs that may result in amputation in people with diabetes. This should empower healthcare professionals with the information and confidence to make a referral for specialist care, which may be the GP, specialist diabetes (or high-risk) podiatry team (in primary or secondary care), the multidisciplinary foot care team, or a walk-in centre or if out-of-hours an emergency facility such as A&E. Note that this is not an exhaustive or definitive list, so the local diabetes referral pathway should be consulted.

The acronym ACT NOW (Figure 31.1) was devised (with direct input from a person with diabetes) to be a safety net for people with diabetes, their carers and healthcare professionals alike, and has been designed to be used with the minimum of training, in all clinical or social settings. The checklist (Figure 31.2) is designed to be used for all people with a foot problem, and the infographic (Figure 31.3) is suitable for those with mental health problems, learning difficulties or dementia and those for whom English is a second language to enable people with diabetes, their carers and healthcare professionals with the tools to ACT NOW (Robbie 2021).

Public Health England (2020) reported that there were 7545 major amputations in people with diabetes in England between 2015 and 2018, with one in three people with diabetes experiencing a foot ulcer during their lifetime (Edmonds et al. 2020). Improved foot care knowledge, assessment and urgent referral, with practical information, is essential as many of the serious complications of foot problems associated with diabetes could be avoided if they were effectively detected, and rapidly assessed, referred and treated at initial presentation in order to ensure the best outcome (Phillips and Mehl 2015).

The ACT NOW checklist (Figure 31.2) was created by a multidisciplinary team of health professionals and a person with diabetes and therefore provides a resilient safety net for high-risk patients by reducing potential delays that may result in poor morbidity outcomes (in terms of ulcer healing and amputations).

iDEAL Group (2020) recommends that the assessment tool should be used for all people with diabetes who present:
- with any foot problem
- by all practitioners
- in all locations

and
- that the initial foot assessment should be in primary or community care
- with urgent referral made to the multidisciplinary foot care team if required.

The ACT NOW assessment tools are designed to be readily available. Use of these resources will ensure consistency in clinical foot assessment (irrespective of which healthcare professional undertakes it) as the individual clinician's skill and judgement regarding the need for escalation to a specialist centre will be the result of a structured clinical history and examination, as well as their own experience. This could ultimately lead to a 50% reduction in major amputations in people with diabetes within five years (Edmonds et al. 2020).

The adoption and regular use of the ACT NOW checklist can maintain the focus on the vital nature of assessment and the need for education, knowledge and awareness to expedite timely referral to save limbs and lives. All healthcare professionals, in both primary and secondary care, have a pivotal role to play in reducing the number of major amputations by adopting ACT NOW and using it routinely (Edmonds et al. 2020).

References

Edmonds, M., Phillips, A., Holmes, P. et al. (2020). To halve the number of major amputations in people living with diabetes, 'ACT NOW'. *Diabetes Prim. Care* 22 (6): 1–5.

iDEAL Group (2020). iDEAL Group Position Statement: ACT NOW! Diabetes and Foot Care Assessment and Referral. https://idealdiabetes.com/publications (accessed 30 October 2020).

Phillips, A. and Mehl, A. (2015). Diabetes mellitus and the increased risk of foot injuries. *J. Wound Care* 24 (5): 4–7.

Public Health England (2020). Diabetes foot care profiles: annual update 2020. www.gov.uk/government/statistics/diabetes-foot-care-profiles-annual-update-2020 (accessed 23 November 2020).

Robbie, J. (2021). Managing foot care for people with diabetes. *Practice Nursing* 32 (Suppl 3): S3–S7.

32 Types of ulcers and their presentations

Figure 32.1 Neuropathic ulcer (after debridement). *Source:* Edmonds et al. 2014 / with permission of John Wiley and Sons.

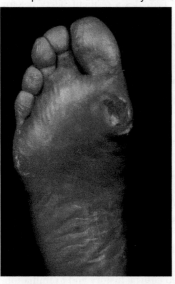

Figure 32.2 Ischaemic ulceration (showing overlying tissue necrosis). *Source:* Edmonds et al. 2014 / with permission of John Wiley and Sons.

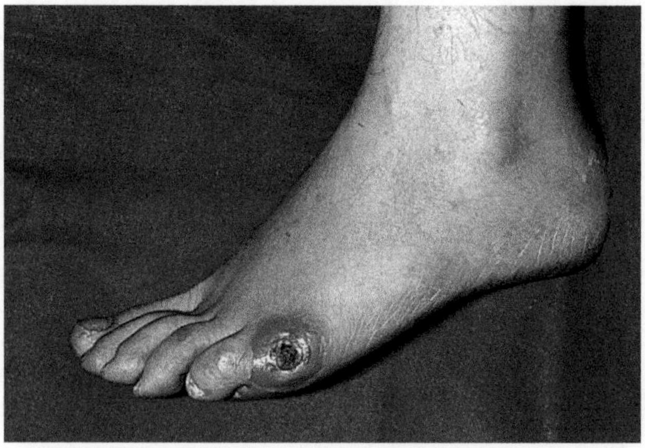

Figure 32.3 Infection is common in all types of ulceration, often spreading rapidly through the foot and resulting in major tissue destruction. *Source:* Edmonds et al. 2014 / with permission of John Wiley and Sons.

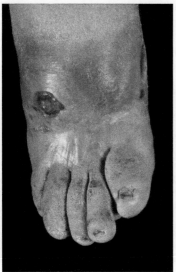

Figure 32.4 The speed at which an infection can evolve in the neuropathic foot and the ischaemic foot. *Source:* Edmonds et al. 2014 / with permission of John Wiley and Sons.

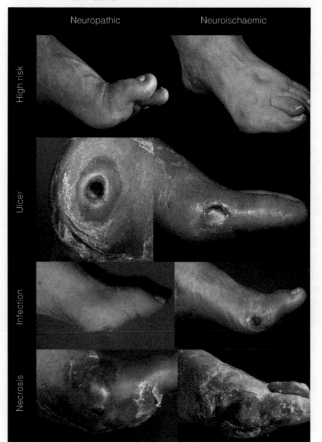

Diabetes Care at a Glance, First Edition. Edited by Anne Phillips.
© 2023 John Wiley & Sons Ltd. Published 2023 by John Wiley & Sons Ltd.

Table 32.1 Comparison of neuropathic and ischaemic ulceration.

Neuropathic ulceration	Ischaemic ulceration
Generally good blood supply Limb/foot usually warm/pink Strong 'bounding' pulses	Evidence of peripheral vascular disease Limb/foot may be cool/pale Weak or absent pulses
Occur on weight-bearing area (plantar foot/dorsal toes/heel)	Occur often on margins of feet or distal toes
Often associated with high foot pressures and overloading	May be associated with trauma
'Punched-out' appearance	Shallow with well-defined border
Often painless	Often painful
Halo of surrounding callus	No callus
May be sloughy or granulating wound bed	May have a necrotic wound bed and/or overlying eschar
Often excessive exudate	Often minimal exudate
May be macerated	No maceration
Requires multidisciplinary team referral for optimal diabetes control and offloading	Requires urgent referral to vascular team for potential vascular surgical intervention to optimize blood flow

Source: Adapted from TeachMe Surgery (2020).

It is an unfortunate statistic that one in three people with diabetes will experience a foot ulcer during their lifetime (Edmonds et al. 2020). This chapter illustrates the different types of ulcerations associated with diabetes and the common complication of infection. There are predominantly two types of foot ulcers in diabetes.

1 Neuropathic ulcers, which occur in patients with loss of peripheral pain sensation (Figure 32.1).
2 Ischaemic ulcers, which occur in people with deficient blood supply to the extremities (Figure 32.2).

The main differences between these two types of ulceration are detailed in Table 32.1. It should be noted that some people may have a combination of both presentations in the form of neuro-ischaemic ulceration.

Infection is common across all types of ulceration, often spreading rapidly through the foot and resulting in major tissue destruction (Figure 32.3). The signs of a red, hot, swollen foot should not be overlooked as progression from an initial minor injury to unsalvageable tissue necrosis and/or overt gangrene can take as little as 48 hours. These red flag markers necessitate the need for rapid referral to a specialist centre for further assessment and treatment:

The acutely red, hot, swollen foot with spreading cellulitis or tracking infection should be referred for urgent antibiotics. If associated with systemic symptoms indicative of sepsis, such as slurred speech or confusion, extreme shivering or muscle pain, breathlessness, an extremely high or a very low temperature, repeated vomiting, seizures, and a rash which does not fade when you press a glass against it (see https://sepsistrust.org/ for further details of signs and symptoms), there is a high indication for hospital admission.

Critical limb ischaemia (Kinlay 2016) is a clinical syndrome of ischaemic pain at rest, with or without tissue loss (such as non-healing ulcers or gangrene) and is related to peripheral arterial disease. It frequently results in a painful, pale, pulseless foot/limb (Figure 32.4).

In addition, purulent or infected gangrene or any foot/limb with increasing rest pain with absent pulses should also be urgently referred to a specialist centre for treatment as the images in Figure 32.4 illustrate the speed at which an infection can evolve in both the neuropathic and the ischaemic foot. Recognition of this emerging situation is essential so that all healthcare providers are able to make an urgent referral in order to save limbs and avoid amputation. Vas et al. (2018) coined the phrase 'Time is Tissue' to illustrate the point that the faster the infection spreads, the more tissue destruction and loss occurs.

It is therefore vital that all people with diabetes, health professionals and multidisciplinary diabetes foot care teams are educated and empowered in their knowledge of foot care and assessment in order to make speedy and timely onward referrals as required and can provide relevant and practical clinical information in order to support the request for specialist intervention to ensure the best outcome for the patient and to avoid the risk of amputation.

References

Edmonds, M.E. and Foster, A.V.M. (2014). *Managing the Diabetic Foot*, 3e. Oxford: Wiley Blackwell.

Edmonds, M., Phillips, A., Holmes, P. et al. (2020). To halve the number of major amputations in people living with diabetes, 'ACT NOW'. *Diabetes Prim. Care* 22 (6): 1–5.

Kinlay, S. (2016). Management of critical limb ischemia. *Circ. Cardiovasc. Interv.* 9(2): e001946. https://doi.org/10.1161/CIRCI NTERVENTIONS.115.001946.

TeachMe Surgery (2020). Lower limb ulcers. https://teachmesurgery. com/vascular/presentations/ulcers (accessed 18 February 2021).

Vas, P.R.J., Edmonds, M., Kavarthapu, V., et al. (2018). The diabetic foot attack: 'Tis Too Late to Retreat!'. *Int. J. Low. Extrem. Wounds* 17(1): 7–13. https://doi.org/10.1177/1534734618755582.

33 Wound healing and tissue viability

Figure 33.1 Phases of wound healing. *Source:* HMP Global, Inc.

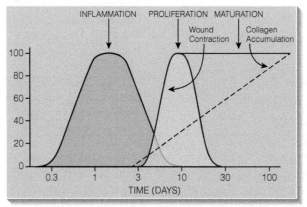

Table 33.1 Wound healing classification.

Primary (first) intention	Secondary (second) intention
No tissue loss	Open wound with tissue loss
Skin edges held together (by sutures, clips, etc.)	Skin edges apart
Healing progresses beneath surface, e.g. surgical sutured wound	Healing occurs by granulation and wound contraction, e.g. wound debridement

Table 33.2 Wound type.

Acute wound	Progresses through the four stages of wound healing without complications, healing within four weeks
Chronic wound	Any wound that has been present for over four weeks and does not progress normally through the stages of healing (often getting 'stalled' in one phase)

Source: Wound Source/HMP Global, Inc.

Wound healing and tissue viability in the context of wounds associated with diabetes is a complex process and identifying the factors that may impede healing is essential in order to plan the appropriate intervention, because inappropriate wound care can significantly contribute to delayed wound healing and poorer patient outcomes.

There are four stages of wound healing: haemostasis, inflammation, proliferation and maturation (Table 33.1) (Wallace et al. 2015). Although the stages of wound healing are sequential, wounds can resolve or deteriorate depending on internal and external patient factors (Schoukens 2009).

1 *Haemostasis* occurs immediately after an injury as the body initiates processes that prevent blood loss to maintain blood pressure and conserve blood volume, with blood vessels constricting to restrict flow. Then, platelets aggregate in order to plug the break in the blood vessel wall. This all happens very quickly as platelets adhere to the endothelial lining within seconds of the rupture of a blood vessel's epithelial wall. Finally, coagulation occurs as blood is transformed from liquid to gel via the release of prothrombin and the first fibrin strands begin to adhere, forming a mesh to reinforce the platelet plug. The formation of a thrombus or clot keeps the platelets and blood cells in the wound area.

2 The *inflammatory phase* is the second stage of wound healing and begins immediately after the injury when the injured blood vessels leak a *transudate* (composed of water, salt and protein) that causes localized swelling. Inflammation both controls bleeding and prevents infection by initiating the repair process and dealing with any bacteria that may be present. During the inflammatory phase damaged cells, harmful cells (pathogens) and bacteria are removed from the wound area (by phagocytosis) and swelling, heat, pain and redness are commonly seen during this stage of the healing process. Inflammation is a natural part of the wound healing process and is only problematic if prolonged or excessive.

3 The *proliferative (reconstruction) phase* comprises epithelialization, angiogenesis, granulation tissue formation and collagen deposition, which enables the wound to contract as new tissue is laid down and the signs of inflammation recede. Myofibroblasts (specialized cells identifiable by smooth muscle within their cytoplasm) are typically found in granulation tissue and scar tissue (fibrosis). They facilitate wound contraction by pulling the wound edges together. In normal wound healing, granulation tissue is pink or red and uneven in texture and will help to heal the wound before epithelial cells resurface the injury (Figure 33.1). It is important to remember that epithelialization (the process

responsible for restoring an intact epidermis) happens faster when wounds are moist and hydrated but not wet.

4 The *maturation (remodelling) phase* occurs when collagen is remodelled to enable full wound closure and is characterized by re-epithelialization, wound contraction and connective tissue reorganization. During the maturation phase, collagen fibres become realigned along tension lines and lie closer together and cross-link, which reduces scar thickness and improves skin strength over time. Generally, remodelling begins about 21 days after an injury and can continue for a year or more.

It should be noted that the stages of wound healing are a complex and fragile process and that failure to progress in these stages can lead to the development of a chronic wound (Table 33.2). Careful wound care will optimize healing by keeping wounds moist and protected to avoid the risk of further injury and/or infection (Jones 2005; Ruben 2016).

Factors that can lead to delayed wound healing include ageing, circulatory disease, local or systemic infection, diabetes, medication (including immunosuppressants and some anti-inflammatories), nutritional deficiencies, stress and smoking.

Diabetes delays wound healing in a number of ways. Hyperglycaemia can prevent necessary nutrients and oxygen from reaching the site of injury, can prevent the immune system from functioning efficiently and increases inflammation in the body's cells, all of which will delay the wound healing process.

Peripheral sensory neuropathy can cause delayed wound healing in people with diabetes as they can continue to injure a wound due to the loss of the protective pain sensation. Peripheral vascular disease results in a reduction of blood flow, which also affects the ability of red blood cells to pass through vessels. Additionally, higher-than-normal blood glucose levels will increase the viscosity (thickness) of blood, further affecting blood flow and delaying healing.

References

Jones, J. (2005). Winter's concept of moist wound healing: a review of the evidence and impact on clinical practice. *J. Wound Care* 14 (6): 273–276. https://doi.org/10.12968/jowc.2005.14.6.26794.

Ruben, B.E. (2016). Clearing the air about moist vs. dry wound healing. Wound Source. https://www.woundsource.com/blog/clearing-air-about-moist-vs-dry-wound-healing.

Schoukens, G. (2009). Bioactive dressings to promote wound healing. In: *Advanced Textiles for Wound Care* (ed. S. Rajendran), 114–152. Cambridge: Woodhead Publishing https://doi.org/10.1016/B978-0-08-102192-7.00005-9.

Wallace, H.A., Basehore, B.M. and Zito, P.M. (2015). Wound healing phases. Last updated 15 November 2021. StatPearls (Internet). https://www.ncbi.nlm.nih.gov/books/NBK470443.

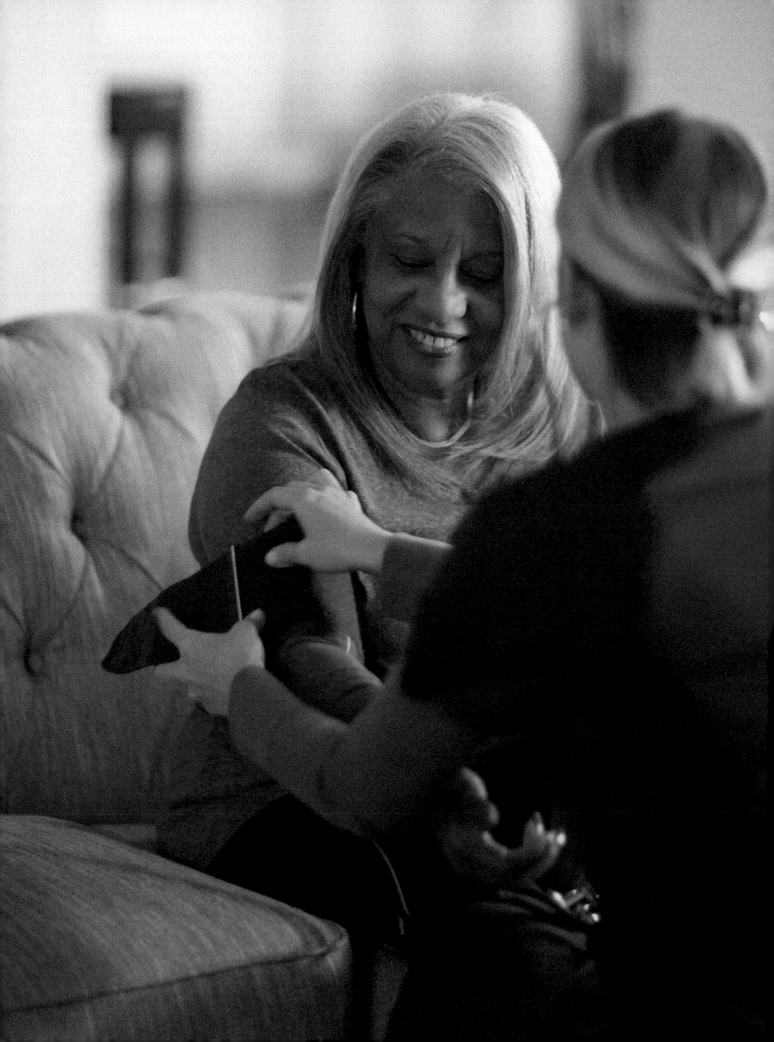

Risk reductions

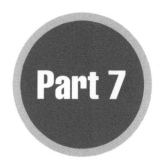

Part 7

Chapters

34 Cardiovascular disease risk reduction

Figure 34.1 Stages of CVD and plaque formation.

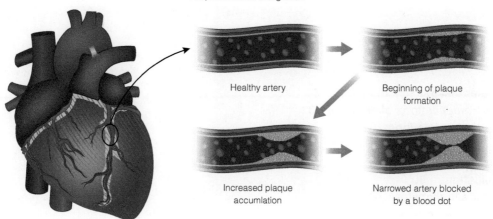

Atherosclerosis stages
Plaque formation and growth

Healthy artery

Beginning of plaque formation

Increased plaque accumlation

Narrowed artery blocked by a blood dot

Figure 34.2 CVD risk factors. *Sources:* Nikolai Titov/Adobe Stock, Vector Tradition/Adobe Stock, lemonaredass/Adobe Stock, elenabsl/Adobe Stock, Favebrush/Adobe Stock, and backup_studio/Adobe Stock.

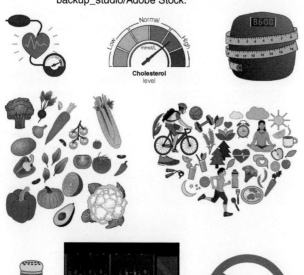

Figure 34.3 Specific targets in people with diabetes.

Blood pressure <140/80 mmHg
In presence of microalbuminuria aim for <130/70 mmHg

Total cholesterol <4 mmol/l

High-density lipoprotein (HDL) cholesterol: at least 1.0 mmol/l in males or 1.2 mmol/l in females

Low-density lipoprotein (LDL) cholesterol: <2.0 mmol/l

HbA1c 48 mmol/mol

Unless risk factors are present, such as older age, frailty, risk of falling, living alone or hypoglycaemic unaware, an individualized target of 53–58 mmol/mol can be agreed with the person concerned

Figure 34.4 UKPDS effects on blood pressure and cholesterol.

Benefits of Tight BP and Tight Glucose Control *UKPDS*

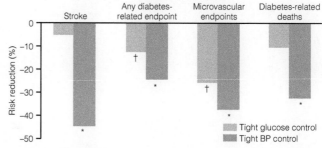

*$P<0.02$, tight BP control (achieved BP 144/82 mm Hg) vs.. less tight control (achieved BP 154/87 mm Hg)
†$P<0.03$, intensive glucose control (achieved HbA$_{1c}$ 7.0%) vs. less intensive control (achieved HbA$_{1c}$ 7.9%)
UKPDS Group. *BMJ.* 1998;317:703-713.
UKPDS Group *Lancet.* 1998,352:837-853.

Cardiovascular disease (CVD) is the term used to describe a group of disorders of the heart and blood vessels caused by atherosclerosis (plaques on the lining of the blood vessels) and thrombosis (blood clots) (Figure 34.1). CVD includes coronary heart disease, stroke, peripheral arterial disease and aortic disease.

CVD is the main cause of death in people with type 2 diabetes and the aim of care for these individuals is CVD risk factor reduction. The overall aims of treatment for CVD is to prevent a cardiovascular event such as a myocardial infarction (heart attack), cerebrovascular event (stroke) or an aortic aneurysm. The approach is to reduce modifiable risk factors through screening, lifestyle advice and medication management.

The risk of CVD is higher in males, in people with a family history of CVD and from populations with certain ethnic backgrounds such as South Asian. CVD risk is higher in people over 50 years old and increases with age; people aged over 85 years are at particularly high risk (National Institute for Health and Care Excellence [NICE] 2016). The risk of CVD is further increased in people with type 1 and type 2 diabetes, and therefore the CVD risk reduction approach is applicable and appropriate for everyone with diabetes from diagnosis. Even in people with optimally controlled CVD risk factors, those with type 2 diabetes still have a 21% higher risk of CVD compared with people without diabetes (Wright et al. 2020).

However, the use of CVD risk calculators has a place in diabetes prevention and can be a useful assessment tool to motivate individuals at risk of diabetes or with pre-diabetes (see Chapter 1) (Figure 34.2). In England and Wales, the QRISK2 Risk Calculator (www.qrisk.org/) is recommended by NICE (2016) and the JBS3 Calculator (www.jbs3risk.co.uk/pages/risk_calculator.htm) is endorsed by the Joint British Societies for the prevention of cardiovascular disease. The JBS3 calculator can estimate short-term risk (10 years) and also lifetime risk. It also contains additional risk factors such as chronic kidney disease (stage 3 or above), migraine, corticosteroid use, systemic blood pressure and sexual dysfunction. In Scotland, the ASSIGN CVD risk assessment (www.assign-score.com/estimate-the-risk/) is recommended by the Scottish Intercollegiate Guideline Network (SIGN 2017).

Risk calculators are not required in people who are at higher risk of CVD, but these can be a useful way to demonstrate to an individual during a consultation what their risk actually is and how much their risk can be potentially reduced by making some modifiable lifestyle changes. Risk calculators are not recommended for use with people with type 1 diabetes or people with established CVD or chronic kidney disease stage 3 or higher (estimated glomerular filtration rate [eGFR] <60 ml/min per 1.73 m^2).

Everyone at risk of CVD should be advised to make lifestyle modifications, which may include diet modifications (increasing fruit and vegetable consumption, reducing saturated fats and dietary salts), increasing physical exercise, sleeping at least eight hours per day, weight management, reducing alcohol consumption and not smoking (Figure 34.2). At the diabetes annual review (see Chapter 29) lifestyle modification, medication review and risk factor modification can be discussed with the use of information prescriptions for individual goal setting as required (see Chapter 10).

Medication approaches include hypertension (blood pressure) management and lipid-lowering medications. In people with diabetes, lower specific targets are used to reduce CVD risk (Figure 34.3). Antiplatelet therapy with low-dose aspirin or clopidogrel for those intolerant of aspirin should only be offered to people with established atherosclerotic disease (NICE 2016). People with diabetes at risk of CVD can experience mood and anxiety disorders, with consideration given to counselling and selective serotonin reuptake inhibitors (SSRIs).

The United Kingdom Prospective Disease Study (UKPDS) and 10-year follow-up study (Holman et al. 2008) demonstrated conclusively that hypertension control and lipid control in diabetes reduces CVD risk above glycaemic control (Figure 34.4). Therefore, CVD risk reduction strategies need to begin at the diagnosis of type 2 diabetes. In type 1 diabetes, CVD risk reduction must also be included in treatment decision-making.

References

Holman, R., Paul, S., Bethel, M. et al. (2008). Long-term follow-up after tight control of blood pressure in type 2 diabetes. *N. Engl. J. Med.* 359 (15): 1565–1576. https://doi.org/10.1056/NEJMoa0806359.

National Institute for Health and Care Excellence (2016). Cardiovascular Disease: Risk Assessment and Reduction, Including Lipid Modification Guideline. NICE Clinical Guideline CG181. Available at www.nice.org.uk/guidance/cg181 (accessed 10 April 2022).

SIGN (2017). Risk Estimation and the Prevention of Cardiovascular Disease. Scottish Intercollegiate Guidelines Network Clinical Guideline 149. Available at www.sign.ac.uk/our-guidelines/risk-estimation-and-the-prevention-of-cardiovascular-disease/.

Wright, A., Suarez-Ortegon, M., Read, S. et al. (2020). Risk factor control and cardiovascular event risk in people with type 2 diabetes in primary and secondary care. *Circulation* 142 (20): 1925–1936. https://doi.org/10.1161/CIRCULATIONAHA.120.046783.

35 Neuropathic complications of diabetes

Figure 35.1 Causes of peripheral neuropathy.

- Obesity and high triglycerides double the risk of diabetes-related peripheral neuropathy.
- Smoking can increase the risk by as much as 42%.
- Hypertension increases the risk from 11% to 65% in data tracked for 37 000 people with type 2 diabetes (Yang et al. 2015).
- Low levels of 'good' HDL cholesterol and high levels of heart-threatening LDL cholesterol increased risk of peripheral neuropathy by 67% (Yang et al. 2015).

Figure 35.2 Glove and stocking presentation of diabetes-related peripheral neuropathy.

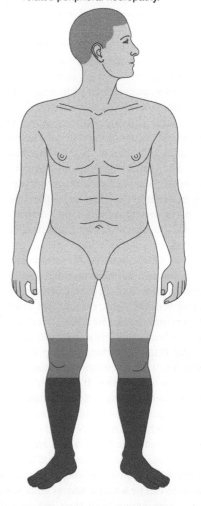

Figure 35.3 Central nervous system, demonstrating the length of the spinal nerves and nerves running from the spinal cord.

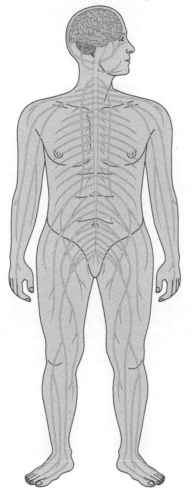

Figure 35.4 Characteristics of neuropathic pain.

- Nocturnal exacerbation (worse at night)
- Hyperaesthesia (excessive physical skin sensitivity)
- Burning/freezing
- Gnawing/aching
- Lancinating jolts of pain
- Dysaesthesia (painful pricking, burning, itching, aching)

Diabetes Care at a Glance, First Edition. Edited by Anne Phillips.

Neuropathic complications affect the nerves and are a microvascular (small-vessel) complication that can occur in people with diabetes. Diabetes-related neuropathy can affect over 90% of people with type 1 and type 2 diabetes (Schreiber et al. 2015). Diabetes is the leading cause of peripheral neuropathy worldwide. Peripheral neuropathy in diabetes causes damage to nerves that lie near to the skin and is caused by suboptimal glucose control and hyperglycaemia (high blood glucose). Other major causes are obesity and high triglyceride levels, smoking, hypertension, and low levels of high-density lipoprotein (HDL) cholesterol (Figure 35.1). Diabetes-related peripheral neuropathy can affect the feet and hands in a glove and stocking presentation (Figure 35.2) and can also affect nerves in the arms and legs.

Nerves are typical cells, as effectively a single cell passes from the brain to the spinal cord and a single cell passes from the spinal nerve root to the skin receptors and can be over 1 m in length. The longest nerves are the most difficult to repair (Figure 35.3), hence the glove and stocking presentation (Figure 35.2).

The commonest presentation is known as distal sensorimotor neuropathy, which presents in a number of ways. The primary presentation comprises sensory losses causing unfelt damage to the foot due to lack of sensation and subsequent ulceration. Neuropathic pain can also be manifest, which is extremely painful and can cause significant disability (Figure 35.4). People should undergo an annual check of their feet for sensory loss (see Chapters 29 and 30), because sensation is protective against ulceration. Neuropathic pain is unusual and hard to describe so assessment tools such as the McGill pain pathway might be useful for assessing an individual's pain (Javed et al. 2015). Neuropathic pain is often resistant to commonly prescribed analgesia; interestingly, some centrally acting medications, including antidepressants such as amitriptyline and anticonvulsants such as gabapentin, can offer some relief. These medications need careful and slow titration and reassessment at regular intervals.

Autonomic neuropathy affects the autonomic nervous system, which controls many bodily functions such as heart rate (Yang et al. 2015) and redirection of blood flow (e.g. shutting down the peripheral circulation when cold and increasing it when hot). The commonest presentations of autonomic dysfunction are sexual dysfunction (see Chapter 41) and dizziness causing postural hypotension that can lead to fainting, in particular when getting out of bed. At annual review (see Chapter 29) measurement of blood pressure sitting and standing is a good diagnostic test for postural hypotension in people with diabetes. Disturbances can also occur in gastrointestinal functioning, known as gastroparesis.

Gastroparesis affects the vagus nerve and alters normal digestion. This can present as discomfort caused by delayed emptying of the stomach and the person affected can vomit; the bowel can also be affected, causing constipation or diarrhoea and sometimes incontinence. This affects glycaemic control and needs referral to a specialist diabetes team for management. Sometimes the bladder can be affected, causing urinary retention and overflow incontinence, and repeated urinary tract infections can trigger this presentation.

Sometimes autonomic neuropathy can influence the usual warning signs of a myocardial infarction (MI) (heart attack) and individuals can experience a 'silent MI' (Yang et al. 2015). Nerve damage can reduce an individual's perception of pain, including the painful presentation of an MI. Despite the high incidence of MI in people with diabetes, most cases will go unnoticed because of diabetes-induced decreased pain sensation due to autonomic neuropathy; these will not receive medical attention and earlier deaths occur (Fokoua-Maxime et al. 2021).

Understanding of people's reactions is required when dealing with those presenting with any of these signs and symptoms and on referral to specialist services such as neurologists, diabetes specialist teams, podiatrists and cardiologists.

References

Fokoua-Maxime, C., Lontchi-Yimagou, E., Cheuffa-Karel, T. et al. (2021). Prevalence of asymptomatic or 'silent' myocardial ischemia in diabetic patients: protocol for a systematic review and meta-analysis. *PLoS One* 16 (6): e0252511. https://doi.org/10.1371/journal.pone.0252511.

Javed, S., Petropoulos, I.N., Alam, U., and Malik, R.A. (2015). Treatment of painful diabetic neuropathy. *Ther. Adv. Chronic Dis.* 6 (1): 15–28. https://doi.org/10.1177/2040622314552071.

Schreiber, A., Nones, C., Reis, R. et al. (2015). Diabetic neuropathic pain: physiopathology and treatment. *World J. Diab.* 6 (3): 432–444. https://doi.org/10.4239/wjd.v6.i3.432.

Yang, C.-P., Lin, C.-C., Li, C.-I. et al. (2015). Cardiovascular risk factors increase the risks of diabetic peripheral neuropathy in patients with type 2 diabetes mellitus: the Taiwan Diabetes Study. *Medicine (Baltimore)* 94 (42): e1783. https://doi.org/10.1097/MD.0000000000001783.

36 # Nephropathic complications

Figure 36.1 Causes of chronic kidney disease.

Diabetes
High glucose levels over time damage the small blood vessels feeding the filtering units in the kidney. Having diabetes for a long time increases the risk of kidney disease.

Hypertension
High blood pressure causes structural damage to the kidneys but also kidney damage causes high blood pressure. Aim for 130/70 mmHg or lower.

Glomerulonephritis
A group of diseases that cause inflammation and damage to the kidney's filtering units. These disorders are the third most common cause of kidney disease.

Polycystic kidney disease
Inherited disease, such as polycystic kidney disease: causes multiple large cysts to form in the kidneys and damage the surrounding tissue.

Infections.
They result from bacteria in the bladder that transfer to the kidneys. Kidney infections are more common in women than in men, as well as in women who are pregnant.

Obstructions.
It usually occurs when an obstruction prevents urine from leaving the kidney. In time the kidney might atrophy, or shrink.

Medications.
Using certain pain medications over a long period of time might result in chronic analgesic nephritis, for example non-steroidal anti-inflammatory drugs (NSAIDs).

Figure 36.2 Risk factors for chronic kidney disease.

- Having diabetes or high blood pressure
- High blood pressure
- Being overweight
- Family history of kidney failure

Figure 36.3 What are the stages of chronic kidney disease?

Stage	Description	eGFR	Kidney Function
1	Possible kidney damage (e.g. protein in the urine) with normal kidney function	90 or above	90–100%
2	Kidney damage with mild loss of kidney function	60–89	60–89%
3a	Mild to moderate loss of kidney function	45–59	45–59%
3b	Moderate to severe loss of kidney function	30–44	30–44%
4	Severe loss of kidney function	15–29	15–29%
5	Kidney failure	Less than 15	Less than 15%

Figure 36.4 Test eGFR if any of these symptoms are present.

Urinating more or less often than usual

Itching

Feeling tired

Swelling in the feet, arms or legs

Muscle cramps

Nausea and vomiting

Loss of appetite

Figure 36.5 Stages of diabetes nephropathy.

Preclinical phase

Stages 1–3 are possible, normal kidney function

Clinical phase

Stage 4: overt proteinuria/clinical nephropathy

Stage 5: end-stage kidney failure

Diabetes is a common cause of chronic kidney disease (CKD), and around 40% of people with diabetes eventually develop diabetic kidney disease (National Institute for Health and Care Excellence [NICE] 2021). The kidney removes toxins and waste products, the most common being urea and creatinine, but many other substances need to be eliminated.

The kidneys act as very efficient filters for eliminating these waste substances, and for returning vitamins, amino acids, glucose, hormones and other vital substances to the bloodstream. The kidneys control acid–base balance – the maintenance of the correct concentration of electrolytes, such as potassium and sodium, and of pH in the extracellular fluid – which is central to homeostasis and thus the effective functioning of all the cells in the body.

The kidneys maintain water balance by regulating the volume of urine they produce, which is influenced by the level of hydration: more urine is produced when fluid intake is high, and less when the body is dehydrated. The kidneys also maintain tight control of the concentrations of electrolytes by returning some to the circulation and excreting excess into the urine.

The kidneys secrete a number of important hormones into the bloodstream. For example, renin is involved in blood pressure control; if blood pressure falls, renin is secreted by the kidneys to constrict the small blood vessels, thereby increasing blood pressure. Erythropoietin is also secreted by the kidney and acts on the bone marrow to increase the production of red blood cells (erythropoiesis). The kidneys also produce an activated form of vitamin D that regulates calcium and phosphate balance, which is essential for healthy bone growth.

There may be no symptoms to indicate that an individual has CKD, so routine screening in people with diabetes is important. As the condition progresses, waste products that are usually filtered by the kidney (e.g. toxins and extra fluid) accumulate in the blood causing uraemia. This can lead to weight loss, poor appetite and nausea, oedema, tiredness and insomnia, haematuria (blood in the urine) and increased need to urinate. Some of the symptoms overlap with other conditions so they are non-specific. Some causes of CKD are shown in Figure 36.1.

Kidney function is usually determined by a measurement known as glomerular filtration rate (GFR). This is time-consuming to measure, so GFR is estimated (eGFR) using a calculation involving blood creatinine concentration, the person's age and other factors. Early-stage kidney disease does not usually cause symptoms, but measurement of eGFR may be recommended if there is higher risk of developing kidney disease (CKD risk factors are shown in Figure 36.2) (KDIGO 2020).

The stages of CKD are described in Figure 36.3. Later-stage CKD can cause symptoms, so eGFR may be requested if any of the symptoms listed in Figure 36.4 are present. Each kidney is composed of filtering units called nephrons, and these can be damaged by high blood glucose levels, with the result that the kidneys filter too much blood. Over time this extra work causes the nephrons to lose their filtering ability. As GFR decreases, this prevents insulin from reaching the cells leading to increased amounts of circulating insulin and therefore to a significant risk of hypoglycaemia.

Diabetic kidney disease (DKD) is characterized physiologically by a decline in eGFR with no or very minimal increase in urine albumin excretion but increasing cardiovascular risk. DKD is seen in both type 1 and type 2 diabetes mellitus but is more common in type 2 diabetes. Diabetic nephropathy (hyperglycaemia-induced glomerular disease) comprises a pattern of gradually rising urine albumin/creatinine ratio (UACR) followed by a steady reduction in eGFR. This represents a protein leak in the capillaries and the protein can be measured in the blood. See Figure 36.5 for the stages of renal failure.

High levels of HbA1c, smoking, high cholesterol, obesity and hypertension increase the risk of diabetic nephropathy in individuals with diabetes. Individuals with a longer duration of diabetes have a higher risk for developing nephropathy. Inadequate glycaemic control is a pivotal risk factor for the development and progression of diabetic nephropathy. Intensive management is essential for preventing and delaying the decline in renal function and progression to diabetic nephropathy.

References

Kidney Disease: Improving Global Outcomes (KDIGO) Diabetes Work Group (2020). KDIGO 2020 clinical practice guideline for diabetes management in chronic kidney disease. *Kidney Int.* 98 (4 Suppl): S1–S115. https://doi.org/10.1016/j.kint.2020.06.019.

National Institute for Health and Care Excellence (NICE) (2021). Chronic Kidney Disease: Assessment and Management. NICE Guidline NG203. www.nice.org.uk/guidance/ng203.

37 Retinal screening

Figure 37.1 Snellen chart.

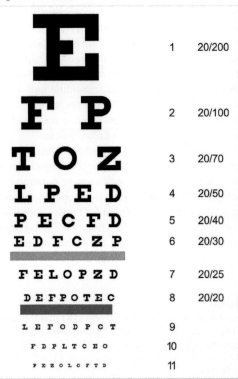

E	1	20/200
F P	2	20/100
T O Z	3	20/70
L P E D	4	20/50
P E C F D	5	20/40
E D F C Z P	6	20/30
F E L O P Z D	7	20/25
D E F P O T E C	8	20/20
L E F O D P C T	9	
F D P L T C E O	10	
P E Z O L C F T D	11	

Figure 37.2 A retinal photograph in diabetic eye screening.
Source: peopleimages.com / Adobe Stock.

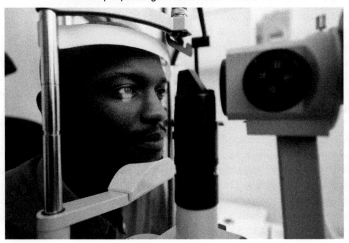

Figure 37.3 Normal retina.

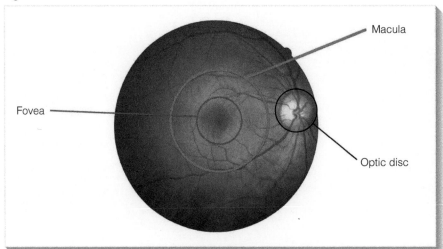

Macula

Fovea

Optic disc

Diabetes Care at a Glance, First Edition. Edited by Anne Phillips.
© 2023 John Wiley & Sons Ltd. Published 2023 by John Wiley & Sons Ltd.

Diabetic retinopathy (DR) is still one of the main reasons for blindness worldwide. This could be due to late presentation for treatment, patient non-attendance at their diabetic services or lack of response to laser and other therapies. Despite great improvements in developing treatments for diabetes care and in laser photocoagulation, along with new advances in eye injections, visual loss remains common.

How does eye screening work? First, the retinal screening service needs an identifiable population and this is provided through referral by the patient's general practitioner (GP), who registers the patient as having diabetes. Once the details are registered with the screening programme, an invitation is issued. The screening test is then performed, and this can be done at a number of locations depending on the patient's preference.

Retinal screeners need to be able to identify eye disease accurately. After the images have been taken, they are assessed and graded. As a result of grading the patient may be referred on for treatment or for closer review or the patient will carry on with their annual check-up, as most screening programmes are performed once a year.

If DR is seen and treatment is considered necessary (see Chapter 38), the screening programme then needs to refer the patient to the hospital eye service for further monitoring or active treatment and this will prevent progression of the eye disease. DR screened and treated at the earliest stage will give optimum results, and the outlook for the condition is good.

At each screening visit the patient will have their visual acuity (VA) checked. VA is a measure of the ability of the eye to distinguish shapes and the details of objects at a given distance. It is important to assess VA consistently in order to detect any changes in vision. One eye is tested at a time. VA commonly refers to the clarity of vision, but technically rates an examinee's ability to recognize small details with precision. VA is dependent on optical and neural factors: (i) the sharpness of the retinal image within the eye, (ii) the health and functioning of the retina, and (iii) the sensitivity of the interpretative faculty of the brain. The most commonly stated VA is far acuity (e.g. 6/6 or 20/20 acuity), which describes the examinee's ability to recognize small details at a far distance (Figure 37.1).

The relevance of measuring the VA is firstly to ensure the VA is stable at each visit, as a reduction in VA could be a surrogate marker for macula oedema (i.e. the build-up of fluid in the macula, an area in the centre of the retina). The retina is the light-sensitive tissue at the back of the eye and the macula is the part of the retina responsible for sharp, straight-ahead vision. Fluid build-up causes the macula to swell and thicken, which distorts vision. VA can also help indicate other conditions, such as significant cataracts, age-related macular degeneration (ARMD) or a central retinal vein occlusion (CRVO). This is performed with a visual occluder and a Snellen chart (Figure 37.1).

Next, the patient's pupils are dilated with tropicamide 1% (remember to warn the person undergoing screening that the drops can sting and feel uncomfortable). Tropicamide inhibits the sphincter pupillae muscle (the strongest muscle in the iris), which stops the pupil contracting and allows clear views and subsequent photographs. After 15–20 minutes the retina is ready to be photographed (Figure 37.2), and two 45-degree images of each retina are taken. In one image the macula is centred and in the other the optic disc is centred. Commonly, two images are taken of each retina, although additional images may be taken to show other areas of pathology (Figure 37.3).

The retinal images are sent for assessment and grading. If any retinopathy is found, a treatment plan is sent to the patient and their GP. The photos are stored for comparison with future screenings. People must be advised not to drive after their pupils have been dilated and to wear sunglasses to avoid the glare of the sun as their vision will be blurry for a few hours after retinal screening until the tropicamide wears off.

It is important for patients with diabetes to undergo retinal screening regularly and they are reminded with a letter to attend. Everyone over the age of 12 years is invited. Good control of diabetes should be encouraged as this will prevent deleterious changes and protect the sight. The screening programme has made a major contribution to the detection and management of retinopathy.

38 Retinopathy

Figure 38.1 R1, background retinopathy: cotton-wool spots (CWS) and haemorrhages are present. This patient would continue with their annual check-ups. No treatment is needed at this stage. *Source:* University hospitals Birmingham NHD Foundation Trust diabetic Retinal Screening Services.

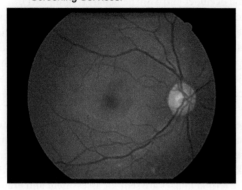

Figure 38.2 R2, pre-proliferative retinopathy: CWS and multiple deep, round or blot haemorrhages are present. This patient would either be referred to the hospital eye service or kept under close review by the diabetic eye screening service (three to six month review). *Source:* University hospitals Birmingham NHD Foundation Trust diabetic Retinal Screening Services.

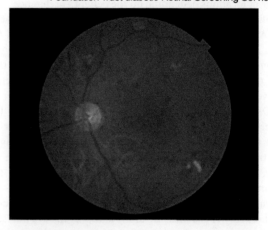

Figure 38.3 R3 NVD: the optic disc shows classic neovascularization. New vessels appear messy in form, tangled and unstable. This patient would need urgent referral to the hospital eye service for anti-VEGF treatment with added laser. *Source:* University hospitals Birmingham NHD Foundation Trust diabetic Retinal Screening Services.

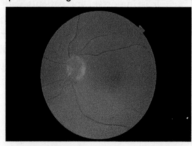

Figure 38.4 R3 NVE plus pre-retinal bleed: haemorrhage occurs from the unstable new vessels bleeding into the internal limiting membrane. Treatment same as above. *Source:* University hospitals Birmingham NHD Foundation Trust diabetic Retinal Screening Services.

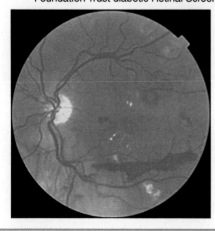

Figure 38.5 M1 maculopathy: characterized by the distribution of exudates, and appearance of yellow waxy deposits of fat. This patient would be referred to the hospital eye service for anti-VEGF treatment. *Source:* University hospitals Birmingham NHD Foundation Trust diabetic Retinal Screening Services.

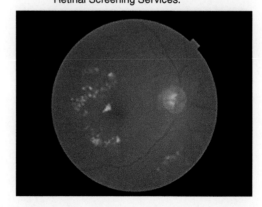

Diabetes Care at a Glance, First Edition. Edited by Anne Phillips.
© 2023 John Wiley & Sons Ltd. Published 2023 by John Wiley & Sons Ltd.

Diabetes is still one of the commonest causes of blindness and some of the ophthalmic complications of diabetes include diabetic retinopathy (DR), earlier development of cataracts, and open-angle and neovascular glaucoma. There is also a higher risk of retinal artery occlusions because of the relation with hypertension (high blood pressure) and hyperlipidaemia (high cholesterol levels), both of which are major modifiable risk factors.

The development of DR arises from damage at the level of the capillaries, the small vessels that run under the retinal bed, resulting in retinal ischaemia and retinal leakage. Each of these breaks down the structure of the blood vessels, and in turn causes problems at the back of the eye. Retinal ischaemia arises from occlusion of a vessel, with the development of cotton-wool spots (Figure 38.1) and then multiple deep haemorrhages and intraretinal microvascular abnormalities, classified as R2 on the national screening protocol (Figure 38.2) and which may proceed to the proliferative stage. If diabetic control is poorly managed and does not improve, conditions in the retina will only deteriorate, and is an indication that the eye will soon be affected by advanced stages.

With capillary closure and neovascularization (R3 NVD; Figure 38.3) and ischaemia, the retina produces vascular endothelial growth factor (VEGF) to compensate for its lack of blood supply. Fortunately, anti-VEGF treatments are available that are useful in the management, while laser treatment will seal leaking blood vessels and reduce the growth. The new vessels are fragile and can bleed into the eye, causing loss of vision (pre-retinal bleed; Figure 38.4), laser treatment will help prevent this.

Retinal leakage is seen as retinal haemorrhages, exudate and oedema. This would be classified as M1 if the changes were seen within the macula (Figure 38.5). Exudate maculopathy occurs due to the release of fats, proteins and water from the retinal capillaries. These are seen as thick, yellow, waxy deposits with sharply defined borders. Maculopathy carries a high risk of loss of central vision, and identifying this sight-threatening disease at the earliest stage will improve the chances of treatment and the long-term outcome. Any exudate within one disc diameter of the fovea should be graded as M1 and referred to hospital eye services; if the visual acuity is affected, an earlier appointment may be needed (Figure 38.5). Treatment of maculopathy can involve a mixture of focal laser and anti-VEGF injections depending on whether it is oedematous or ischaemic; occasionally, both treatments are given as the retina presents both conditions.

Intravitreal injection of drugs has been shown to be an effective and safe means of drug delivery to the retina, and has led to improvements in diabetic maculopathy. Although these drugs act rapidly to reduce retinal oedema, the effects wear off within a few weeks and the eye will require repeat injections. This is why a combination of anti-VEGF injections and laser produce the best long-term results.

Education and feedback for the patient will also benefit the treatment, along with referral to general practitioners, diabetes physicians and optometrists; this flow of information will allow optimal medical management.

39 Liver complications

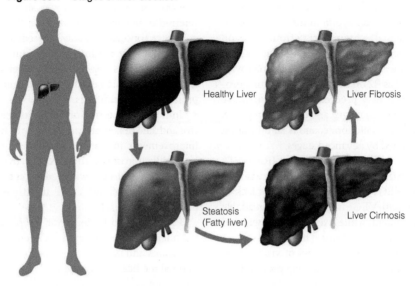

Figure 39.1 Stages of liver disease.

Healthy Liver

Liver Fibrosis

Steatosis
(Fatty liver)

Liver Cirrhosis

Figure 39.2 Stages of liver failure.
Source: British Liver Trust.

Liver failure

healthy liver   fatty liver   fibrosis   cancer

Figure 39.3 Reversible and irreversible liver disease. *Source:* British Liver Trust.

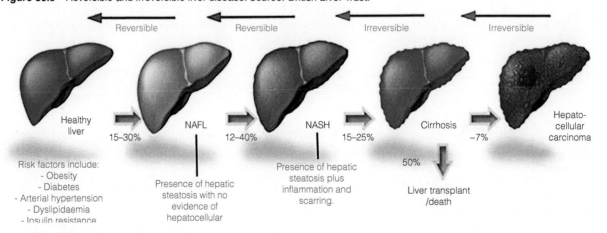

Reversible   Reversible   Irreversible   Irreversible

Healthy liver   15–30%   NAFL   12–40%   NASH   15–25%   Cirrhosis   ~7%   Hepato-cellular carcinoma

Risk factors include:
- Obesity
- Diabetes
- Arterial hypertension
- Dyslipidaemia
- Insulin resistance

Presence of hepatic steatosis with no evidence of hepatocellular

Presence of hepatic steatosis plus inflammation and scarring.

50%

Liver transplant /death

Diabetes Care at a Glance, First Edition. Edited by Anne Phillips.
© 2023 John Wiley & Sons Ltd. Published 2023 by John Wiley & Sons Ltd.

This chapter describes the association between type 2 diabetes and non-alcoholic fatty liver disease (NAFLD) that can cause serious complications for patients with these conditions. The impact of liver disease on the management of diabetes is also discussed. Adams et al. (2010) identified that not only is NAFLD common among patients with type 2 diabetes but that these patients have an increased mortality rate. Patients with type 2 diabetes are at increased risk of their NAFLD progressing to non-alcoholic steatohepatitis (NASH) and an increased risk of cirrhosis and hepatocellular carcinoma (HCC) (Figure 39.1).

NAFLD leads to a build-up of excess lipids (fats) in the liver (Liu et al. 2014). The structural damage produced in the liver is similar to that caused by alcoholic liver disease, but alcohol intake in these patients is minimal. The damage can range from steatosis (fat within the liver cells) to fibrosis (the formation of scar tissue), cirrhosis (a late stage of scarring) and NASH (British Liver Trust 2022) (Figures 39.2 and 39.3). Once decompensated liver failure has occurred, some patients may eventually require a liver transplant (Patel et al. 2016). It is predicted that cirrhosis due to NAFLD will in due course become the leading cause for liver transplantation.

The number of people with NAFLD is increasing and it is very common in patients with type 2 diabetes; it is also increasingly found in people with pre-diabetes and this offers an opportunity for diabetes prevention strategies to be discussed at this point (see Chapter 1). The connection between type 2 diabetes and NAFLD is complex and there are many hypotheses regarding how they are linked. As well as a higher incidence of NAFLD in patients with diabetes, it is clear that patients with NAFLD have a higher risk of developing type 2 diabetes, especially in the later stages of fibrosis; this is independent of other risk factors such as obesity. It has also been observed that if NAFLD improves, then this can reduce the risk of developing type 2 diabetes.

There are no licensed treatments for NAFLD, but trials continue to try to develop these. Some of the trials that have been carried out have included medications used to treat type 2 diabetes. Glucagon-like peptide 1 (GLP-1) agonists reduce blood glucose levels and help with weight reduction in patients with type 2 diabetes. Two research trials using liraglutide and semaglutide (see Chapter 14) concluded that they can reduce hepatic fat and improve NAFLD (Newsome et al. 2021; Armstrong et al. 2016), but as yet these drugs have not been approved as a treatment for NAFLD.

At present, diet and lifestyle changes continue to be the only recommended treatment for NAFLD; this also has a positive effect on type 2 diabetes so can have multiple positive benefits. A previous review of a multidisciplinary team clinic, consisting of hepatologists, diabetes consultant, specialist nurse and specialist liver dietitian, demonstrated the benefits of this combined approach in patients with NAFLD (Armstrong et al. 2014). The use of sodium/glucose cotransporter (SGLT) inhibitors has also been shown to have benefits in some trials.

Managing patients with type 2 diabetes and liver disease can be difficult, since many treatments developed for type 2 diabetes have limited evidence and safety for use in patients with liver disease and this is reflected in the available guidance. Monitoring diabetes in these patients is also difficult. HbA1c has limitations: in cirrhosis, HbA1c can be lower, though plasma glucose levels are not affected and this could lead to misdiagnosis or underestimation of a patient's glucose control.

The literature also suggests that patients with cirrhosis can develop insulin resistance, leading to difficulties in controlling blood glucose levels, and insulin is therefore used more frequently in these patients. Initially, insulin requirements will be high; however, as the liver disease progresses the patient's requirements can reduce and therefore close monitoring is important.

Overall the management of patients with liver disease and diabetes is very difficult. The limited research available for the treatments and the impact on HbA1c poses a challenge for all involved and close monitoring with a multidisciplinary team is beneficial.

References

Adams, L., Harmsen, S., St Sauver, J. et al. (2010). Non-alcoholic fatty liver disease increases risk of death among patients with diabetes: a community-based cohort study. *Am. J. Gastroenterol.* 105 (7): 1567–1573. https://doi.org/10.1038/ajg.2010.18.

Armstrong, M.J., Hazlehurst, J.M., Parker, R. et al. (2014). Severe asymptomatic non-alcoholic fatty liver disease in routine diabetes care; a multi-disciplinary team approach to diagnosis and management. *QJM.* 107: 33–41.

Armstrong, M.J., Gaunt, P., Aithal, G.P. et al. (2016). Liraglutide safety and efficacy in patients with non-alcoholic steatohepatitis (LEAN): a multicentre, double-blind, randomised, placebo-controlled phase 2 study. *Lancet.* 387: 679–90.

British Liver Trust (2022). NAFLD, NASH and fatty liver disease. Available at https://britishlivertrust.org.uk/information-and-support/living-with-a-liver-condition/liver-conditions/non-alcohol-related-fatty-liver-disease.

Liu, Y., Reeves, H., Burt, A. et al. (2014). *TM6SF2* rs58542926 influences hepatic fibrosis progression in patients with non-alcoholic fatty liver disease. *Nat. Commun.* 5: 4309. https://doi.org/10.1038/ncomms5309.

Newsome, P., Buchholtz, K., Cusi, K., et al. (2021). A placebo-controlled trial of subcutaneous semaglutide in non-alcoholic steatohepatitis. *N. Engl. J. Med.* 384: 1113–1124. https://doi.org/10.1056/NEJMoa2028395.

Patel, Y., Berg, C. and Moylan, C. (2016). Non-alcoholic fatty liver disease: key considerations before and after liver transplantation. *Dig. Dis. Sci.* 61(5): 1406–1416. https://doi.org/10.1007/s10620-016-4035-3.

40 Skin conditions in diabetes

Figure 40.1 Acanthosis nigricans. *Source:* Brady et al. 2017 / StatPearls Publishing LLC / CC BY 4.0.

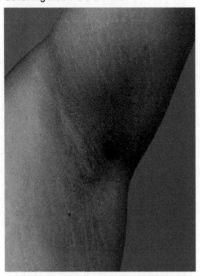

Figure 40.2 Necrobiosis lipoidica diabeticorum. *Source:* Richard et al., 2010 / with permission from John Wiley & Sons.

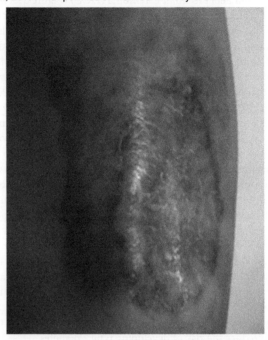

Figure 40.3 Lipohypertrophy at injection sites.

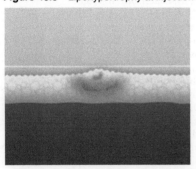 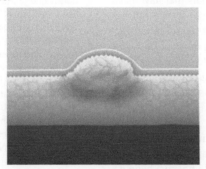 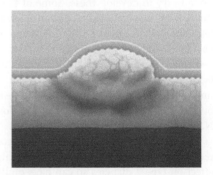

Figure 40.4 Vitiligo. *Source:* Andrii / Adobe Stock.

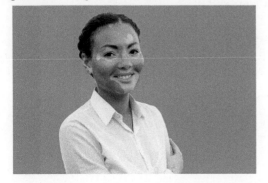

Figure 40.5 Disseminated granuloma annulare. *Source:* Mierlo / Wikimedia Commons / Public Domain; SreeBot / Wikimedia Commons / CC BY-SA 2.0.

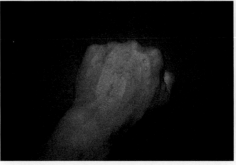 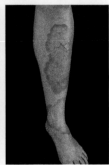

Diabetes Care at a Glance, First Edition. Edited by Anne Phillips.
© 2023 John Wiley & Sons Ltd. Published 2023 by John Wiley & Sons Ltd.

Diabetes mellitus is a common and complex disorder that can affect a variety of organs including the skin. It has been estimated that between 30 and 70% of people with diabetes mellitus, regardless of type, may present with a skin condition at some point during their lifetime (Labib et al. 2022).

Acanthosis nigricans

Acanthosis nigricans is a fairly common condition and appears as a darkening of the skin in skin folds, frequently the neck, armpits, groin and joints such as of the fingers and toes (Figure 40.1). The skin becomes velvety to the touch, thickened and leathery and the most common cause is being overweight. Other causes include type 2 diabetes or other conditions that affect hormone levels, such as Cushing's disease, polycystic ovary syndrome or an underactive thyroid. Acanthosis nigricans is considered to be a clinical manifestation of insulin resistance (González-Saldivar et al. 2017). While there is no specific treatment for the acanthosis nigricans patches themselves, a dermatologist may be able to suggest treatments to improve their appearance. Finding and treating the cause is usually recommended first and the patches should fade. Depending on the cause, a GP will recommend weight loss and medications for insulin resistance and type 2 diabetes.

Necrobiosis lipoidica diabeticorum

Necrobiosis lipoidica diabeticorum (NLD) is a disorder frequently affecting the shins of people with diabetes, although it can also appear on the hands, forearms and trunk. It is more common in women and causes raised, red, shiny patches (often with a yellow centre and visible blood vessels) (Figure 40.2). It may be itchy and painful where the skin is red and inflamed, which can cause further injury resulting in ulceration. The cause of NLD is not known; it often occurs following a minor injury like a graze or bruise but can appear for no reason. Around half of the people who have NLD also have type 1 diabetes (prevalence <1%). The best way to prevent NLD is to take good care of the skin by using a daily moisturizer, using a neutral soap and by ensuring that skin is thoroughly dried after washing. Use of camouflaging creams can also be useful.

Lipohypertrophy

Lipohypertrophy is a skin disorder that can affect people with diabetes who inject insulin subcutaneously, and is characterized by a series of fatty lumps under the skin that can also feel firm to the touch. They frequently occur when insulin is injected repeatedly in the same place (Figure 40.3). Lipohypertrophy can be easily prevented by rotating injections sites; if it does form, avoiding injections at the affected site for a prolonged period will help it to resolve. If this condition is suspected the person should see their diabetes healthcare team for advice because it reduces the effect of the insulin as it is not absorbed appropriately through the lipohypertrophic lumps.

Fungal skin infections

Fungal skin infections, including thrush and candida infections, often occur in people with diabetes who have elevated levels of glucose in their bloodstream. They are more prone to developing bacterial or fungal skin infections due to potential suppression of their immune system, poor circulation of blood to the skin, loss of feeling (that alerts a person to injury) due to peripheral sensory neuropathy, or the body's high-glucose environment which makes an ideal setting for infection. The most common fungal skin infection is thrush, an unpleasant infection that can occur in the genitals, mouth and armpits. It can be resolved with medication and should be treated as soon as possible as it can be passed between people via physical contact with the infected site. The GP will be able to recommend an appropriate oral antifungal medication such as fluconazole 150 mg and this can also be bought over the counter at pharmacies.

Vitiligo

Vitiligo is much more prevalent in people with diabetes mellitus and occurs more frequently in women (Figure 40.4). It occurs in approximately 1% of the general population, but is more common in people with type 1 than type 2 diabetes mellitus (estimates suggest 1–7% of patients with vitiligo have diabetes) (Gopal et al. 2014). As type 1 diabetes is an autoimmune disease, this tends to support the autoimmune theory of vitiligo, with higher levels of inflammatory cytokines in patients with vitiligo and concomitant type 1 diabetes compared to patients with vitiligo only, which supports the potential inflammatory link between the two conditions. A referral to a dermatologist may be necessary and treatments include corticosteroid creams, laser treatment and light therapy.

Disseminated granuloma annulare

Disseminated granuloma annulare often affects children and young adults with diabetes and presents as rings or arcs on the fingers, hands, feet and ears that may be red, reddish-brown or skin tone (Figure 40.5). These are usually painless although they may itch and usually heal without treatment. For small areas, topical steroids can be a useful treatment option.

Prevention

The best way to prevent skin problems occurring as a result of diabetes is to maintain blood glucose levels within the target range. If a skin condition is suspected, it is vital that the person with diabetes accesses specialist help without delay. The GP may decide to refer to a dermatologist for further tests or may be able to treat the condition without further appointments.

Diligent hygiene is important, with regular washing and careful drying with the use of daily moisturizers (emollients) to hydrate the skin and keep it in optimum condition. If a wound develops, a sterile dressing should be applied to avoid infection developing and specialist advice sought.

References

González-Saldivar, G., Rodríguez-Gutiérrez, R., Ocampo-Candiani, J. et al. (2017). Skin manifestations of insulin resistance: from a biochemical stance to a clinical diagnosis and management. *Dermatol. Ther.* 7 (1): 37–51. https://doi.org/10.1007/s13555-016-0160-3.

Gopal, K.V.T., Raghurama Rao, G., and Kumar, Y.H. (2014). Increased prevalence of thyroid dysfunction and diabetes mellitus in Indian vitiligo patients: a case-control study. *Indian Dermatol. Online. J.* 5 (4): 456–460.

Labib, A., Rosen, J., and Yosipovitch, G. (2022). Skin manifestations of diabetes mellitus. In: *Endotext* [Internet] (ed. K.R. Feingold, B. Anawalt, A. Boyce, et al.). South Dartmouth, MA: MDText.com Inc. Available at https://www.ncbi.nlm.nih.gov/books/NBK481900.

41 Sexual dysfunction in people with diabetes

Figure 41.1 Different types of couples. *Sources:* (top to bottom) peopleimages.com/Adobe Stock, Rido/Adobe Stock and Jacob Lund/Adobe Stock.

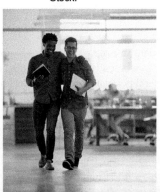

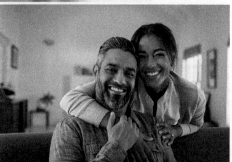

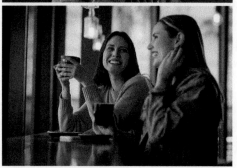

Figure 41.2 Medications that can cause sexual dysfunction.

Drug group	Examples	Usual indication
Beta-blockers	Atenolol, metoprolol, bisoprolol	Angina, acute coronary syndrome, hypertension
Thiazide diuretics	Bendroflumethiazide, chlortalidone	Hypertension, oedema
Anti-androgens	Finasteride	Prostatic disease
Major tranquillizers	Chlorpromazine, flupentixol	Major psychiatric illness
Antidepressants	Fluoxetine	Depression

Figure 41.3 Physical causes of sexual dysfunction in women with diabetes.

Physical cause	Effects
Blood vessel damage caused by atherosclerosis	Vaginal dryness and lack of blood flow to the clitoris affecting orgasm
Neuropathic damage	Reduced sensation, making arousal and orgasm more difficult
Associated endocrine disorders of the pituitary or thyroid gland	Problems with production of hormones which play an important role in normal sex drive. Low levels of these hormones can lead to a loss of sexual interest, desire and function
Low oestrogen levels	Disorders in the production of hormones which affect the amount of lubrication produced during sexual arousal
Smoking, recreational drugs and alcohol	All of these can affect blood flow to the clitoris and disturb messages between the clitoris, vagina and brain before and during sex. This can make orgasm very difficult to achieve

Figure 41.4 A useful questionnaire to use with women to detect sexual dysfunction.

Question (diabetes specific	Rationale
What medications are you currently taking?	To establish whether there are any possible iatrogenic-related influences that can be addressed
Are you experiencing any stress or depressive symptoms?	To review if depression is present and to enable disussion if this is the case. Review of treatment if depression is alredy diagnosed
Have you recently had a baby?	To find out whether the woman has experienced a difficult delivery or birth injuries, and whether she is getting enough sleep and has sufficient support to help her
Do you feel tired all the time?	To establish whether this is the result of hyperglycaemia or hypoglycaemic unawareness, which can both cause fatigue. If the woman's sleep pattern is disturbed, she may be experiencing anxiety, stress or depression
Do you have vaginal dryness?	To find out whether this is related to diabetes control, neuropathy, medication, hormones or the menopause, and whether the woman would like to have treatment for this
Do you feel uncomfortable or experience pain during sex?	To explore whether this may be causing sexual anxiety
Do you have recurrent infections, especially thrush or urine infections?	To investigate whether this is caused by suboptimal control of the diabetes. Fungal infection is easily treatable and advice regarding blood glucose control can be given
Do you feel there is a problem with your relationship with your partner?	To explore whether the woman is experiencing marital tension or guilt about relationships, each of which can inhibit sexual experience
Do you feel embarrassed by the sex act?	To discover whether or not a past negative experience or previous abuse may be influencing the present situation
Do you have a poor self-image?	To give the woman an opportunity to discuss any feelings of depression or low self-esteem, for example as a result of obesity, which can have a negative effect on sexual function
Have you experienced sexual or physical abuse?	To discover whether the woman has had a past negative experience (see above)

Diabetes Care at a Glance, First Edition. Edited by Anne Phillips.
© 2023 John Wiley & Sons Ltd. Published 2023 by John Wiley & Sons Ltd.

Sex is an important part of relationships for all adults of all ages. Sexual dysfunction in men and women is becoming increasingly better recognized as an aspect of living with diabetes. Awareness is growing about the difficulties that female and male sexual dysfunction can cause in relationships. People can experience guilt and rejection, and often depression, which is more common in people with diabetes (Cauwenberghe et al. 2022).

Exploring sexuality and sexual well-being is part of the holistic nature of diabetes care. The needs of people with diabetes who may be experiencing sexual dysfunction, sexual identity problems or complexities with sex need recognition and inclusion in individualized diabetes care (Figure 41.1). Diabetes is thought to double the risk of sexual problems in men and women and sexual dysfunction is more commonly the result of physical and psychological causes.

Erectile dysfunction is defined as the inability to achieve and maintain a penile erection adequate for satisfactory sexual intercourse. Erectile dysfunction can define a full or partial erection but which is insufficient for penetration or fades away before satisfactory intercourse is complete (Defeudis et al. 2022). Erectile dysfunction is 3.5 times higher in men with diabetes than those without and its complications include a sedentary lifestyle and increased body weight.

Erectile dysfunction in men is associated with older age, use of antihypertensive medications (Figure 41.2), smoking, alcohol use, higher body mass index, and severity and duration of diabetes. Cardiovascular and neuropathic complications can also cause abnormalities of endothelial cells, the thin layer of cells that line blood vessels, which in turn leads to abnormalities in blood vessel function. These functional abnormalities are linked with cardiovascular disease and can lead to sexual dysfunction in both men and women. Erectile dysfunction is associated with higher HbA1c levels and lipidaemia. Erectile dysfunction is also linked with a 15-fold increase in coronary heart disease and/or neuropathic complications (Cauwenberghe et al. 2022).

Identifying sexual problems can be more complex in women but is strongly related to physical causes (Figure 41.3) or psychological factors, although the metabolic factors of diabetes do still have an influence. Figure 41.4 offers a useful assessment tool when discussing sexual dysfunction with women. Every factor contributing to normal sexual functioning can be potentially involved in sexual dysfunction. Orgasm, the culmination of sexual arousal, is a reproductive necessity in men, but not in women.

Sexual dysfunction in women can be influenced by a number of causes including physical, lifestyle and relationship factors and the effects of medications (Enzlin et al. 2009). Female sexual dysfunction usually refers to problems with vaginal lubrication and sensation. The four main areas of sexuality that women can experience difficulty with involve desire, arousal, dyspareunia (pain with intercourse) and orgasm. Women may not discuss these issues with their partners because of feelings of frustration, embarrassment and guilt and this can make the problem worse if the cause is unknown.

Decreased blood flow to the clitoris and vagina can result from a number of factors, including cardiovascular disease, atherosclerosis, hypertension, diabetes, dyslipidaemia, prior pelvic trauma or surgery, pelvic fracture, straddle injury, hysterectomy, birth injury, smoking or side effects of medications (Phillips and Phillips 2015).

Embarrassment and guilt can inhibit both men and women from discussing their sexual difficulties; if they are worried their diabetes is implicated, they may find this harder to cope with. Health professionals have a duty of care to offer holistic care to people with diabetes and sexual health and well-being are included within this care.

References

Cauwenberghe, J., Enzlin, P., Nefs, G. et al. (2022). Prevalence of and risk factors for sexual dysfunctions in adults with type 1 or type 2 diabetes: results from Diabetes MILES – Flanders. *Ddiabet. Med.* 39 (1): e14676. https://doi.org/10.1111/dme.14676.

Defeudis, G., Mazzilli, R., Tenuta, M. et al. (2022). Erectile dysfunction and diabetes: a melting pot of circumstances. *Diabetes Metab. Res. Rev.* 38 (2): e3494. https://doi.org/10.1002/dmrr.3494.

Enzlin, P., Rosen, R., Wiegel, M. et al. (2009). Sexual dysfunction in women with type 1 diabetes: long-term findings from the DCCT/EDIC study cohort. *Diabetes Care* 32 (5): 780–785. https://doi.org/10.2337/dc08-1164.

Phillips, A. and Phillips, S. (2015). Recognising female sexual dysfunction as an essential aspect of effective diabetes care. *Appl. Nurs. Res.* 28 (3): 235–238. https://doi.org/10.1016/j.apnr.2015.04.007.

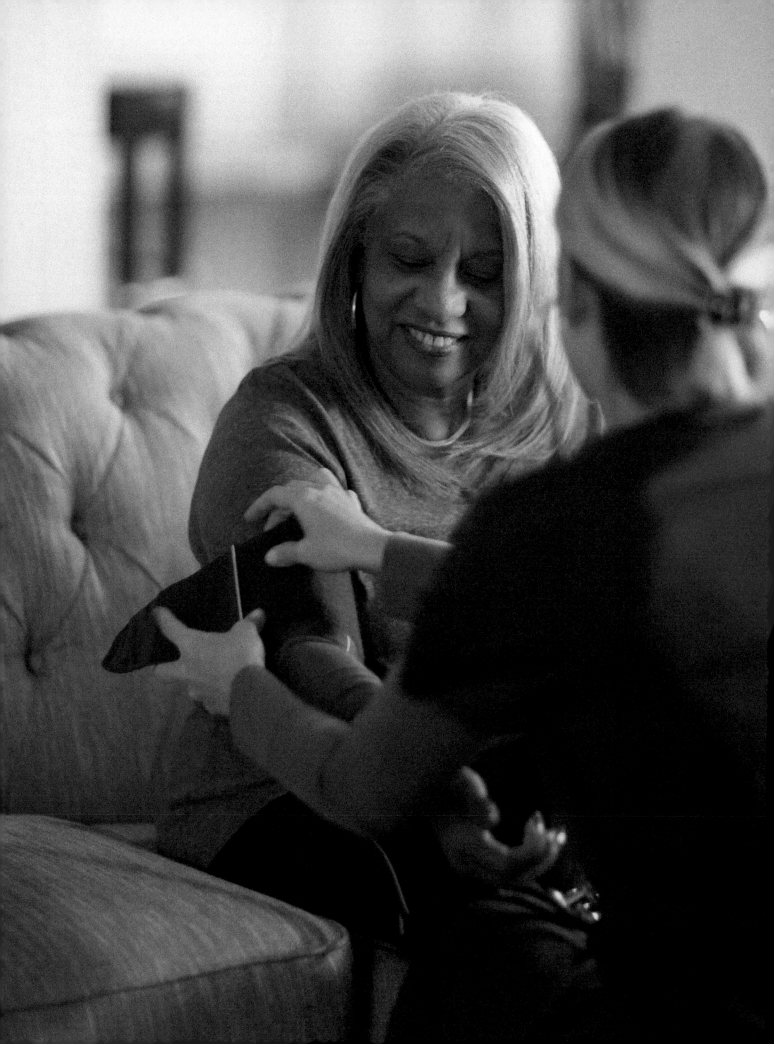

Other considerations

Part 8

Chapters

42 Travel and diabetes

Figure 42.1   Essential general travel advice.

Obtain comprehensive travel insurance and declare you have diabetes: NB Read the small print to check what is covered
Ensure you have over six months still valid on your passport when you plan to travel
Obtain a UK Global Health Insurance Card (UK GHIC) to offer healthcare cover when abroad
Research your destination and be aware of local laws and customs
Tell someone where you are going and leave emergency contact details with him/her
Take enough money and have access to emergency funds
Pack a first aid kit including over the counter medications

Figure 42.2   Diabetes-specific travel advice.

- Pre-order and pack extra supplies or oral medications, blood glucose testing strips and/or insulin
- Carry a current repeat prescription strip in hand luggage for ease of access
- Carry hypoglycaemia treatments in hand luggage in non-liquid from
- Carry insulin or diabetes injectable medications such as glucagon-like peptide- I (GLP-I) in hand luggage only
- Carry extra supplies for insulin administration in hand luggage and within the suitcase. Split the supplies between these in case the suitcase does not arrive at the destination
- Avoid ordering a diabetes-specific meal on the flight as this may be low in carbohydrate
- Pack a cooling wallet to carry insulin if travelling to a warm destination
- Pack and carry emergency contact numbers and travel insurance in hand luggage
- Carry a Medical ID

Figure 42.3   Useful travel websites for advice and information.

- European Health Insurance Card (EHIC) www.ehic.org.uk/Internet/startApplication.do
- NHS Fit 4 Travel www.fitfortravel.nhs.uk/resources/links-to-useful-websites.aspx
- Travel Health Pro http://travelhealthpro.org.uk/
- TRAVAX – Up to date Travel information for Health Professionals www.travax.nhs.uk/
- For further information: National Travel Health Network and Centre www.nathnac.org and in Scotland from Health Protection Scotland www.hps.scot.nhs.uk
- Diabetes UK Travel and Diabetes www.diabetes.org.uk/travel

Figure 42.4   Medications to stop if experiencing vomiting or diarrhoea.

- Metformin
- Angiotensin-converting enzyme (ACE) inhibitors
- Angiotensin II receptor blockers (ARBs)
- Diuretics
- Dipeptidyl peptidase 4 inhibitors
- GLP-1 agents
- Sodium/glucose cotransporter (SGLT2) inhibitors
- These medications can cause dehydration and acute renal failure during vomiting or diarrhoea

Diabetes Care at a Glance, First Edition. Edited by Anne Phillips.
© 2023 John Wiley & Sons Ltd. Published 2023 by John Wiley & Sons Ltd.

An essential requirement for a person with diabetes to travel safely is that adequate planning and preparation must be undertaken before the intended trip. Travel can involve time zone changes and increase the potential risk of infection, which can cause difficulties with glycaemic control. Pre-travel advice should be sought at least four to six weeks before the intended journey and may help to plan for contingences in order to reduce travel-related risks. Figure 42.1 illustrates the essential general travel advice while Figure 42.2 lists diabetes-specific travel advice.

Attention to glycaemic control before travelling can help reduce glucose fluctuations such as hypoglycaemia, hyperosmolar hyperglycaemic state or ketoacidosis, and seeking advice from a health practitioner about medication or insulin dosing is recommended. It should also be suggested that the individual carries a repeat prescription strip with their current prescribed medications and also sick day advice (see Chapter 23) to act as a reminder when unwell or if involved in an accident.

About two-thirds of all travel insurance claims are for medical conditions (Leggat and Zuckerman 2015) and some travel insurance companies may not offer travel insurance to people with diabetes, so travellers with diabetes should be advised to seek insurance early before the trip and to check what is covered. The insurance premiums are likely to be elevated for people with diabetes as their risk is seen as medium to high. People with diabetes are required to purchase comprehensive travel insurance and to declare their diabetes and any associated complications at the time of purchase.

Pre-planning to ensure an adequate supply of insulin or oral medications and other supplies, such as glucose testing strips and a method for checking ketones by blood or urine, is essential. If the individual is using technology such as an insulin pump or continuous glucose or flash glucose monitoring, then spares for all these devices also need including.

Information about the insulin available in other countries can be obtained from pharmaceutical companies, but outside the European Union insulin may only be available in strengths other than the usual U100 prescribed in the UK. Access to insulin may also be difficult in some countries so pre-planning is essential to ensure the individual knows where and how to access insulin in an emergency (Zwar 2018).

Supplies of insulin or other injectable diabetes medication such as glucagon-like peptide 1 (GLP-1) must be carried in hand luggage (the hold on long-haul flights freezes and this can damage insulin). Blood glucose test strips and oral medications (except those needed for the flight) can be placed in the suitcase that will stored in the hold. Because of the increased risk of terrorism, pre-planning and advice about carrying non-liquid glucose sources for hypoglycaemic management in hand language is recommended. The ultimate decision about whether a person can fly safely is the prerogative of each airline, but people with diabetes are likely to be asked to supply a fitness-to-fly letter that documents their need to carry their medical supplies. For older people with comorbidities, a pre-travel health screening is advised.

To avoid a deep vein thrombosis (DVT) during long-haul flights, travellers with diabetes should wear appropriate flight socks of the correct size, undertake leg exercises and maintain hydration (Yagel et al. 2022). Short-haul flights require no adjustment to insulin doses but long-haul flights across time zones will require planning with a health professional. Individuals taking oral medications and/or GLP-1 injectable agents are advised to keep to their normal regimens and adjust to the time zone of their destination upon arrival. The Diabetes UK 'Travel and Diabetes' webpages (Figure 42.3) are very useful resources to help plan a safe and trouble-free trip.

Holidays can cause problems with blood glucose control so having a detailed plan to help cope with sickness or diarrhoea can help prevent an emergency admission while abroad. Travellers' diarrhoea can ruin a holiday or a business trip, with some destinations being at higher risk than others. Figure 42.4 details the medications that should be temporarily stopped during an episode of vomiting or diarrhoea to avoid dehydration and potential acute renal failure. Changes in diet, alcohol consumption and possible water-borne infections (from swimming pools, lakes and rivers) can trigger diarrhoea.

Specific advice about the following should also be sought.

- Sun safety: the increased absorption of insulin due to vasodilation causing hypoglycaemia can be avoided by insulin dose reductions and careful glucose monitoring. At high altitudes there is an increased risk of sun damage so individuals arranging skiing trips or mountaineering holidays need to plan for increased monitoring and reducing insulin doses as required to reduce hypoglycaemia.
- Footwear should be worn at all times to avoid burn injuries from hot swimming pool tiles, especially if someone has neuropathic complications whereby they are unable to detect or feel an injury.
- Insect bites can cause many diseases and the National Travel Health Network and Centre (NaTHNaC) Travel Health Pro website or TRAVAX can be used before travel to check for current outbreaks of diseases and for country-specific advice.

References

Leggat, P. and Zuckerman, J. (2015). Pre-travel health risk assessment. In: *Essential Travel Medicine* (ed. J.N. Zuckerman, G. Brunette and P. Leggat). Oxford: Wiley Blackwell.

Yagel, O., Abbasi, M., Leibowitz, D., and Herzog, E. (2022). Travel related venous thromboembolism. In: *Pulmonary Embolism* (ed. E. Herzog). Cham: Springer https://doi.org/10.1007/978-3-030-87090-4_19.

Zwar, N. (2018). Travelling with medicines in 2018. *Australian Prescriber* 41 (4): 102–104. https://doi.org/10.18773/austprescr.2018.034.

43 Monogenic diabetes

Figure 43.1 Obtaining a family tree can be helpful in discovering monogenic diabetes.

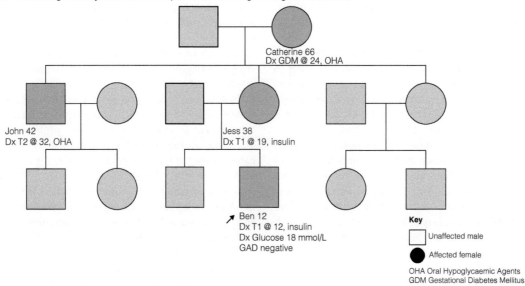

Catherine 66
Dx GDM @ 24, OHA

John 42
Dx T2 @ 32, OHA

Jess 38
Dx T1 @ 19, insulin

Ben 12
Dx T1 @ 12, insulin
Dx Glucose 18 mmol/L
GAD negative

Key

☐ Unaffected male

● Affected female

OHA Oral Hypoglycaemic Agents
GDM Gestational Diabetes Mellitus

Figure 43.2 How to diagnose monogenic diabetes instead of type 1 or type 2 diabetes.

When should a diagnosis of monogenic diabetes be considered rather than type 1 diabetes?

- All patients diagnosed <9 months of age
- Patients diagnosed aged >9 months if islet autoantibodies negative or other features are present (e.g. developmental disorder, unusual family history)
- Family history of diabetes in one parent and other first-degree relatives of that affected parent.
- Absence of islet autoantibodies, especially if measured at diagnosis.
- Preserved beta-cell function, with low insulin requirements and detectable C-peptide (either in blood or urine) over an extended partial remission phase (> 5 years after diagnosis)

When should a diagnosis of monogenic diabetes be considered rather than type 2 diabetes?

- Absence of severe obesity.
- Lack of acanthosis nigricans and/or other markers of metabolic syndrome.
- Family history of diabetes in one parent and other first-degree relatives of that affected parent, especially if any family member with diabetes is not obese.
- Unusual distribution of fat, such as central fat with thin or muscular extremities.

Figure 43.3 Monogenic diabetes.

Clinical findings	Possible diagnosis	Treatment
Mild stable fasting hyperglycaemia which does not progress	Glucokinase (*GCK*)	None required
Renal abnormalities, genital tract abnormalities	*HNF1B*	Insulin
Macrosomia and/or neonatal hypoglycaemia	*HNF4A*	Sulfonylurea (low dose)
Renal glycosuria	*HNF1A*	Sulfonylurea (low dose)

Diabetes Care at a Glance, First Edition. Edited by Anne Phillips.
© 2023 John Wiley & Sons Ltd. Published 2023 by John Wiley & Sons Ltd.

Monogenic diabetes results from a change or deletion in a single gene and accounts for 1–6% of paediatric diabetes cases (Johansson et al. 2017). The disease may be inherited within families as a dominant, recessive or non-Mendelian trait or may present spontaneously as a de novo mutation (i.e. not inherited from parents). Over 40 different genetic subtypes of monogenic diabetes have been identified to date, each having a typical phenotype and a specific pattern of inheritance.

Treatment decisions for monogenic diabetes are based on the individual gene, allowing a specific treatment approach for each person (Johansson et al. 2017). A confirmed diagnosis enables genetic counselling and extended genetic testing in other family members with diabetes or hyperglycaemia who may also carry a pathogenic mutation (Figure 43.1).

All paediatric patients negative for GAD, IA2 and zinc transporter islet autoantibodies should be considered for genetic testing for monogenic diabetes. Preventing a delay in the correct molecular diagnosis of patients can improve treatment and quality of life and reduce treatment and monitoring costs (Figure 43.2).

Maturity-onset diabetes of the young (MODY) affects 1–2% of people with diabetes (1–3% of those aged under 30 years), although it often goes unrecognised. The three main features of MODY are as follows.

- Diabetes develops before the age of 25 years.
- Diabetes runs in families from one generation to the next (although sporadic de novo mutations may occur).
- Low or no insulin requirements more than five years after diagnosis (stimulated C-peptide >200 pmol/l or >0.2 nmol/mmol if urine C-peptide/creatinine ratio [UCPCR]) and lack of typical type 2 characteristics (increased body mass index, acanthosis nigricans) (Hattersley et al. 2018).

MODY runs in families because of a change in a single gene involved in the development or function of beta cells; it is passed on by affected parents to their children, termed autosomal dominant inheritance. All children of an affected parent with MODY have a 50% chance of inheriting the affected gene and developing MODY themselves. Absence of islet autoantibodies and modestly raised glucose at diagnosis are critical features of MODY (lower HbA1c and absence of diabetic ketoacidosis). The most common MODY diagnoses involve the genes GCK, HNF1A, HNF4A and HNF1B. More genes remain to be identified (see https://www.diabetesgenes.org/tests-for-diabetes-subtypes/a-new-test-for-all-mody-genes).

A detailed past medical and family history, as well as an individual diabetes history (glucose and ketones at diagnosis, islet autoantibodies), are useful for indicating what the specific diabetes diagnosis may be (Figure 43.3). The MODY calculator developed in Exeter indicates how likely the person is to have MODY and can be found at https://www.diabetesgenes.org/exeter-diabetes-app/. Referral to a specialist in monogenic diabetes or an interested clinical genetics unit is recommended where predictive or pre-symptomatic testing of asymptomatic individuals is requested.

Establishing the correct molecular diagnosis of MODY avoids misdiagnosis as type 1 or type 2 diabetes and, depending on the specific diagnosis, may allow more appropriate treatment and more accurate prognosis of the risk of complications. It may avoid stigma and limitation of employment opportunity (especially in the case of GCK) and enables prediction of risk in a first-degree relative (unless it is a de novo mutation) or in an offspring (Hattersley et al. 2018).

Neonatal diabetes mellitus (NDM) diagnosed before six months is rare (approximate incidence 1 in 100 000 live births) and reflects severe beta-cell dysfunction. It is most likely to have a monogenic cause rather than being due to autoimmunity (Edghill et al. 2006). There are many different subtypes of NDM, defined by different genetic causes. Currently, genetic testing finds a genetic diagnosis for over 80% of patients with neonatal diabetes. Approximately half will require lifelong treatment to control hyperglycaemia – permanent neonatal diabetes mellitus (PNDM). Some have a potassium channel mutation (KCNJ11 and ABCC8) and can be treated with high-dose sulfonylureas. Others have transient neonatal diabetes mellitus (TNDM), which will resolve within a few weeks or months but may later relapse (often in teens/young adulthood). In addition, the diagnosis will inform other likely features, for example developmental delay and epilepsy.

Type 1 diabetes (T1D) is a polygenic autoimmune disease. Patients with T1D may develop other autoimmune conditions (e.g. coeliac disease, autoimmune hypothyroidism/ hyperthyroidism). There may be a strong family history of autoimmunity due to a shared polygenic risk (HLA genes in particular).

However, a mutation in a single gene can cause autoimmune diabetes, likely to be diagnosed as T1D. Approximately half have islet autoantibodies and usually no measurable C-peptide. These patients often have many other autoimmune disorders (e.g. immunodysregulation, polyendocrinopathy, enteropathy, X-linked, termed IPEX syndrome) and are generally diagnosed under the age of two years. Their complexity can make management challenging. Immunosuppression specific for each genetic subtype may be beneficial but haematopoietic stem cell transplant is currently the only curative treatment for monogenic autoimmunity.

There is increasing recognition of heterogeneity in T1D with immunological overlap between monogenic subtypes and some patients with T1D, leading to the possibility of the development of targeted treatment interventions for T1D in the future.

References

Edghill, E.L., Dix, R.J., Flanagan, S.E. et al. (2006). HLA genotyping supports a nonautoimmune etiology in patients diagnosed with diabetes under the age of 6 months. Diabetes 55 (6): 1895–1898.

Hattersley, A.T., Greeley, S.A.W., Polak, M. et al. (2018). ISPAD Clinical Practice Consensus Guidelines 2018: The diagnosis and management of monogenic diabetes in children and adolescents. Pediatr. Diabetes 19 (Suppl 27): 47–63.

Johansson, B.B., Irgens, H.U., Molnes, J. et al. (2017). Targeted next-generation sequencing reveals MODY in up to 6.5% of antibody-negative diabetes cases listed in the Norwegian childhood diabetes registry. Diabetologia 60 (4): 625–635.

44 Older people with diabetes

Figure 44.1 Dry eyes. *Source:* ia_64/Adobe Stock.

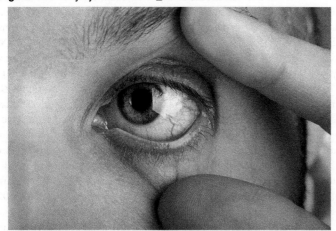

Figure 44.2 Dry skin.

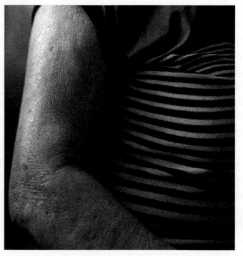

Figure 44.3 Frailty and diabetes. *Source:* Andrey Bandurenko / Adobe Stock.

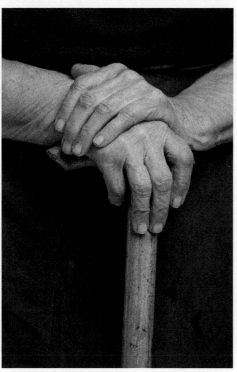

Figure 44.4 Polypharmacy is a risk for hypoglycaemia. *Source:* Mediteraneo/Adobe Stock.

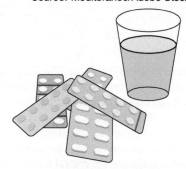

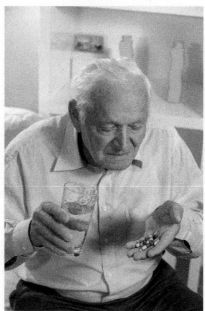

The presentation and management of diabetes in older people can be complicated by existing comorbidities, shortened life expectancy and the amplified consequences of adverse effects due to antidiabetes treatments. Older adults are more prone to hypoglycaemia and are at risk of these consequences in relation to falls, fractures and cardiovascular events, which increase all-cause mortality.

Diabetes is more common in older adults as beta cells naturally wear out and reduce in number and effectiveness of insulin production as we age. Abnormal glucose tolerance is present in about 60% of adults over 60 years of age as the beta-producing insulin cells in the islets of Langerhans in the pancreas decline, and insulin sensitivity increases with age. Older people with type 2 diabetes may not present with the usual symptoms of polydipsia (excessive thirst), polyuria (excessive urination) or polyphagia (excessive hunger). The renal threshold for glucose also increases with age so glycosuria may not be detected.

The presentation of diabetes can be altered, so practitioners need to be aware of assessing and taking into consideration those presenting with dehydration with altered thirst perception and delayed fluid supplementation. Keratoconjunctivitis sicca (dry eyes; Figure 44.1), xeroderma (dry skin; Figure 44.2), confusion (see Chapter 45), unhealing wounds like leg ulcers, pressure sores or urinary tract infections can also occur. Increased bone fractures and the increased presence of frailty syndrome indicate potential undiagnosed diabetes (Figure 44.3).

After diagnosis, evidence suggests that overtreatment of older adults with diabetes is common, with many having experienced treatment intensifications in previous years in order to meet National Institute for Health and Care Excellence (NICE) guidance targets. Additionally, any recent hospitalization can result in treatment escalation due to subsequent hyperglycaemia. Furthermore, if the older person is now relying on carers to help with taking medications and with meal preparation or following admission to a residential or nursing home, this can dramatically improve HbA1c levels due to regular nutrition and access to medication. Regular review and attention to de-escalation of antidiabetes therapies, such as shorter-acting insulins or sulfonylureas, is opportune to reduce risk of hypoglycaemia.

Frailty is common with diabetes, and this increases risk on the individuals affected. Frailty is described as 'a condition characterized by a loss of biological reserves across multiple organ systems and vulnerability to physiological decompensation after a stressor event' (Clegg et al. 2013). There are several ways to evaluate frailty using assessments such as the electronic Frailty Index (eFI) (https://www.england.nhs.uk/ourwork/clinical-policy/older-people/frailty/efi). This assesses the patient's health records and presenting symptoms against set criteria and if 36 deficits are recorded, then frailty is diagnosed. However, clinical judgement is equally important. Prognosis and appropriate treatment goals need to vary according to the individual presentation of the older person and need to be personalized to aim to keep the individual as safe as possible and reduce risk optimally. For example, older and more frail people have numerous comorbidities and develop and experience cognitive decline and can be more dependent on others. They are at increased risk from hypoglycaemia and therefore Strain et al. (2021) advise aiming for HbA1c levels of 59–64 mmol/mol in these individuals. Regular medication review and review of renal function are advised, as declining renal function can precipitate increased episodes of hypoglycaemia (Alsahli and Gerich 2015). Monitoring of HbA1c is pivotal in older people as this prompts treatment review, especially if insulin resistance has subsided or weight has decreased, which often occurs in older adults. Reducing the pill burden and simplifying the prescription can make medication taking much easier to manage (Figure 44.4).

The assessment of frailty should be a routine part of diabetes reviews for older people, following which the quality of life, glycaemic targets and therapeutic choices can be modified accordingly. Strain et al. (2021) suggest that frailty is a dynamic process that may be improved by removal of hyperglycaemia and hypoglycaemia.

References

Alsahli, M. and Gerich, J. (2015). Hypoglycaemia in patients with diabetes and renal disease. *J. Clin. Med.* 4 (5): 948–964. https://doi.org/10.3390/jcm4050948.

Clegg, A., Young, J., Iliffe, S. et al. (2013). Frailty in elderly people. *Lancet* 381: 752–762.

Strain, D., Dawn, S., Brown, P. et al. (2021). Diabetes and frailty: an expert consensus statement on the management of older adults with type 2 diabetes. *Diabetes Ther.* 12 (5): 1227–1247.

45 Cognitive decline and diabetes

Figure 45.1 Cognitive decline and dementia. *Source:* freshidea/Adobe Stock.

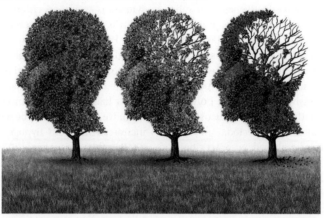

Figure 45.2 Alzheimer's disease and vascular dementia.

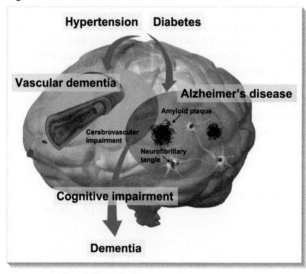

Figure 45.3 Symptoms of vascular dementia.

Slowness of thought

Difficulty with planning and understanding

Problems with concentration

Changes to mood, personality or behaviour

Feeling disorientated and confused

Difficulty walking and keeping balance

Symptoms of Alzheimer's disease as many people with vascular dementia also have Alzheimer's disease.

Figure 45.4 Treatments.

Eating a healthy, balanced diet

Losing weight if overweight

Stopping smoking

Getting fit

Cutting down on alcohol consumption

Taking medications to treat hypertension, hyperlipaemia or to prevent blood clots.

Physiotherapy

Occupational therapy

Memory Cafes

Psychological therapies

Diabetes Care at a Glance, First Edition. Edited by Anne Phillips.

Globally, cognitive decline leading to dementia has become one of the most common disabling conditions in all societies. The numbers of people diagnosed with dementia are doubling every 20 years, with predictions of 75.6 million in 2030 and 135.5 million by 2050 (Xue et al. 2019). The population trends for dementia and cognitive decline are mirroring those for diabetes and considerable overlap exists in the risk factors and pathophysiological processes (Arnold et al. 2018). There are over 200 different types of dementia, usually diagnosed at over 65 years of age. The most common types are Alzheimer's, vascular dementia, dementia with Lewy bodies, frontotemporal dementia and mixed dementia (Dementia 2017).

Cognitive decline and dementia can be classified by their presentation and presenting signs (Figure 45.1). The presence of vascular dementia is increased in type 2 diabetes and is related to type 2 being closely associated with cardiovascular diseases. Individuals with type 2 diabetes show an accelerated cognitive decline, specifically identifiable in executive function and information processing awareness. Younger onset of type 2 diabetes is also linked with a higher risk of dementia. Insulin resistance in the brain is connected with a reduced ability to use glucose to fuel normal brain functions.

Hyperglycaemia causes a dramatic increase in beta-amyloid peptide and one of the symptoms of Alzheimer's disease is the production and deposition of beta-amyloid peptide in the brain (Figure 45.2). Alzheimer's disease is a progressive neurological disorder that causes the brain to shrink (atrophy) and brain cells to die. This is the most common dementia, and it causes a continuous decline in thinking and behavioural and social skills that affects a person's ability to live independently. The mortality rate in Alzheimer's disease usually ranges from 3 to 10 years post diagnosis; however, with type 2 diabetes this is accelerated to three to six years. Untreated vascular complications such as hypertension are associated with a faster rate of progression.

Vascular dementia is by far the most common form in people with diabetes. People with vascular dementia live for around five years after the onset of symptoms, as vascular dementia shares the same risk factors as heart attacks and strokes, and these are the most usual causes of death. Vascular dementia can start very suddenly or develop slowly over time. Symptoms are shown in Figure 45.3. Causes of vascular dementia include diabetes, hypertension, stroke, mini-strokes (known as transient ischaemic attacks), smoking and being overweight.

There is no current cure for vascular or any other dementias. Treatment is aimed at reducing the progression of cognitive decline and encouraging people affected to undertake activities, as outlined in Figure 45.4.

Type 1 diabetes increases the risk of dementia by 93%. The link appears to be an association with glucose control and fluctuating glucose management, from high (hyper) to low (hypo) glucose levels. In hyperglycaemia, concentration, memory and thinking processes can be impaired. In hypoglycaemia (glucose <4 mmol/l), confusion can reduce the ability to make decisions safely and impairs brain function due to lack of glucose for brain metabolism.

In individuals with dementia, hypoglycaemia should be avoided; keeping glucose levels high can help prevent the risks of hypoglycaemia for people who cannot communicate that their glucose levels are dropping. This is particularly important for people in the later stages of dementia when aphasia (difficulty in speaking) can occur, as the individual will be unlikely to communicate their needs effectively. Because hypoglycaemia may present as 'uncharacteristic behaviour', it may be perceived as deteriorating mental status and thus missed. As the glucose level decreases, the individual is at risk of falls, losing consciousness or choking and this can trigger complications such as heart attacks or stroke. All health professionals and carers need to know how to recognize and treat hypoglycaemia (see Chapter 22) to keep people with diabetes and dementia safe.

References

Arnold, S.E., Arvanitakis, Z., Macauley-Rambach, S.L. et al. (2018). Brain insulin resistance in type 2 diabetes and Alzheimer's disease: concepts and conundrums. *Nat. Rev. Neurol.* 14: 168–181. www.nature.com/articles/nrneurol.2017.185.

Dementia UK (2017). Types and symptoms of dementia. www.dementiauk.org/about-dementia/types-of-dementia/.

Xue, M., Xu, W., Ou, Y.-N. et al. (2019). Diabetes mellitus and risks of cognitive impairment and dementia: a systematic review and meta-analysis of 144 prospective studies. *Ageing Res. Rev.* 55: 100944. https://doi.org/10.1016/j.arr.2019.100944.

46 End of life and diabetes

Figure 46.1 Trend Diabetes *End of Life Guidance for Diabetes Care*.

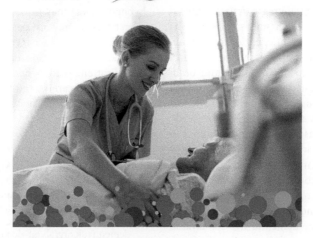

Figure 46.2 End-of-life care. *Source:* Joel bubble ben / Adobe Stock.

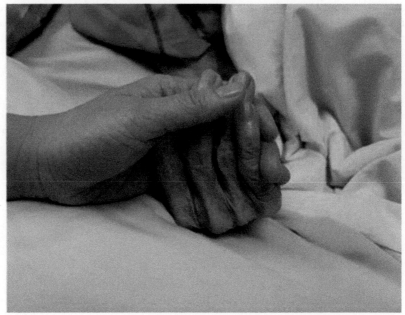

Diabetes is one of the most common comorbidities in end-of-life care, with approximately 10% or more of people dying having diabetes. The majority of people with diabetes will not be dying directly due to diabetes but it is likely to complicate the management of their care. Diabetes can also be the result of diabetogenic treatments, such as the use of steroids.

Throughout a person's life, if diabetes has been present then there has most likely been a plan, goals and medication to optimize diabetes management in order to prevent both microvascular and macrovascular complications. At the end of life, in the last year, months, weeks or days there needs to be a change of emphasis – there needs to be a plan to optimize quality of life.

There is no research or evidence base to support a particular blood glucose range. However, according to experts (Trend Diabetes 2021) (Figure 46.1) the recommendation for a person who is coming to the end of their life, on medication that may cause hypoglycaemia (i.e. insulin and/or sulfonylureas), is that glucose levels should be between 6 and 15 mmol/l. However, it is important to consider the individual and their wishes; having discussions to explain new potential targets and the risk of hypoglycaemia is important.

For people with type 2 diabetes, the end of life often comes with reduced appetite, anorexia and sometimes nausea and vomiting. Often diabetes medication can be reduced and/or stopped. Sulfonylureas can cause hypoglycaemia so should be reduced or stopped if glucose levels are not too high. Glucagon-like peptide 1 (GLP-1) is not normally recommended in end of life due to its appetite-reducing and weight-loss effects. Sodium/glucose cotransporter 2 (SGLT2) inhibitors are also not recommended due to their adverse effect on fluid balance and the risk of diabetic ketoacidosis (DKA) in people who are acutely ill or not eating. Medication that is given to prevent longer-term complications, such as statins, angiotensin-converting enzyme (ACE) inhibitors or aspirin, can also be stopped.

For people with type 1 diabetes, insulin should be continued to reduce the risk of DKA, although towards the last days of life a simpler, once or twice daily long-acting/background insulin can be used on its own. In type 2 diabetes, insulin can normally be reduced and stopped depending on glucose control, as individuals should not be at risk of DKA because people with type 2 diabetes still produce some of their own insulin.

Hypoglycaemia should be avoided in end-of-life care. Hypoglycaemia can be distressing and also difficult to treat when people may have difficulty eating or have a reduced appetite. This is why the target for end of life is a minimum glucose level of 6.0 mmol/l, well above the hypoglycaemia threshold. Insulin or sulfonylureas should be reduced if a person is experiencing hypoglycaemia or glucose level is continually below 6.0 mmol/l.

Steroid therapy is regularly used in palliative and end-of-life care. Steroids stimulate the liver to release glucose and therefore in people with diabetes they can cause hyperglycaemia; in people without diabetes they can cause steroid-induced hyperglycaemia. The hyperglycaemia can cause osmotic and distressing symptoms so needs treating. The typical glucose profile is for the glucose levels to rise during the day but then drop overnight. In people who are not on diabetes medication, morning gliclazide or morning isophane insulin often works well. People already on diabetes treatment are likely need to need intensification. Seeking advice from the diabetes team is recommended.

Towards the end of life appetite is often reduced. This may impact diabetes control, especially for people on quick-acting/mixed insulin that should be given with food; they may need to change to a longer-acting insulin that does not need to be given with food. In type 2 diabetes, a reduced appetite and weight loss will most likely require a de-escalation of therapy. At this stage, people with type 2 diabetes can frequently come off their diabetes medication. It should also be noted that metformin tends to reduce appetite and may cause gastrointestinal side effects so it may be appropriate to reduce or stop this medication too.

People with diabetes may have restricted what they eat in the past as a way of treating their diabetes and it is therefore important at this time to encourage a pleasure-related diet and discuss how having smaller, but higher-calorie food can be beneficial as well as improving quality of life.

In the very last days of life (Figure 46.2), further de-escalation of therapy is required and should ideally be planned for. If the person has type 2 diabetes and on diet or diet and oral medications, the medications can be stopped and there is no need to continue glucose monitoring. For people with type 2 diabetes on insulin, insulin should be stopped if on a small amount and glucose level less than 10 mmol/l.

If on larger amounts of insulin, the insulin dose can be reduced by at least 25% of the total daily dose and changed to a long-acting once or twice daily insulin. The glucose level can be checked just once a day in the late afternoon; if the glucose level is less than 8.0 mmol/l, the insulin dose can be reduced by 10–20%. If glucose level is greater than 20.0 mmol/l, the insulin dose can be increased by 10–20%.

For people with type 1 diabetes, insulin should be continued but just once or twice daily long-acting insulin. Again, the glucose can be checked just once a day in the afternoon. If the glucose level is less than 8.0 mmol/l, the insulin dose can be reduced by 10–20%. If glucose level is greater than 20.0 mmol/l, the insulin dose can be increased by 10–20%.

It should be noted that when someone is dying, ketones are likely to be produced due to not eating and fatty acid breakdown, but this is not DKA. In addition, due to peripheral shutdown, capillary blood glucose may give a falsely low reading.

In summary, good palliative and end-of-life care requires planning and good communication. When a person has diabetes this needs to be included. Open and honest communication and explanation will help to ensure that the focus is on quality of life, and reducing the risk of acute complications and related symptoms of diabetes.

Reference

Trend Diabetes (2021). End of Life Guidance for Diabetes Care. Available at https://diabetes-resources-production.s3.eu-west-1.amazonaws.com/resources-s3/public/2021-11/EoL_TREND_FINAL2_0.pdf

Index

Diabetes Care at a Glance, First Edition. Edited by Anne Phillips.
© 2023 John Wiley & Sons Ltd. Published 2023 by John Wiley & Sons Ltd.